Does This Pregnancy Make Me Look Fat?

Does This Pregnancy Make Me Look Fat?

Claire Mysko and Magali Amadeï

Health Communications, Inc.
Deerfield Beach, Florida

www.hcibooks.com

Library of Congress Cataloging-in-Publication Data

Mysko, Claire.
   Does this pregnancy make me look fat? : the essential guide to loving your body
before and after baby / Claire Mysko and Magali Amadeï.
      p.   cm.
   ISBN-13: 978-0-7573-0792-8
   ISBN-10: 0-7573-0792-2
   1. Pregnant women—Health and hygiene. 2. Pregnancy—Psychological aspects.
3. Body image in women. 4. Beauty, Personal. I. Amadeï, Magali. II. Title.
   RG525.M97 2009
   618.2—dc22   2009028272

Publisher: Health Communications, Inc.
            3201 S.W. 15th Street
            Deerfield Beach, FL 33442–8190

Cover design by Justin Rotkowitz
Interior design by Lawna Patterson Oldfield
Interior formatting by Dawn Von Strolley Grove
Interior illustrations ©Monica Martinez

Some names of those interviewed have been changed to protect their privacy.

Contents

The Healthy Beauty Pledge
for Mothers and Mothers-to-Be

I promise to . . .

Acknowledge that there is no such thing as the "perfect" body—or the "perfect" mommy.

Never define my self-worth according to the number on the scale or the size of my clothes.

Make decisions that are right for me. They don't have to be right for everyone else.

Ask for help when I need it. I'll make a phone call, write an e-mail, or send a text—whatever it takes to reach out for support.

Take care of myself and take time for myself, even if some days I can only manage one-minute increments.

Separate the retouched, made-up beauty fantasies in the media from what matters most to me in reality.

Work on developing a relationship with food that is about health, nourishment, and enjoyment, not deprivation, indulging, and punishment.

Stop all body-bashing talk with my friends, my colleagues, my partner, my family, and myself.

Give up the mission to get my "prebaby body" back and start focusing my energy on moving *forward* in my new life.

Remember that, one person at a time, healthy beauty is a revolution—for ourselves and for our children.

Signed _____

Introduction

Let's get something out of the way right now. This book will not tell you how to get your prebaby body back. But don't stop reading yet. Instead, consider if you can relate to any of the following scenarios: A group of female colleagues meet for lunch. When the half-eaten grilled chicken salads are cleared from the table, they agonize over which dessert to share. A fudge brownie plus three spoons adds up to fifteen minutes of discussion about who thinks she's carrying a little extra weight these days and who can't believe she's being so "bad" by indulging. In a shop downtown, one friend gives another a pep talk through a dressing-room door, offering heartfelt reassurances that it's the fluorescent lights—not her thighs—that are the problem. On the other side of town, a pregnant woman sits in the waiting room of her obstetrician's office. Surrounded by tabloid magazines and pamphlets for Botox, she tries to steel herself for the moment she's been dreading all week: stepping on the scale.

As women, we are well-schooled in the language of weight loss and weight gain. Turn on your TV and count the minutes until you see a diet-related commercial. Log on to Facebook and you might find yourself staring at a muffin top ad or a quiz to determine if you are a certifiable lard ass. There is, to put it simply, a lot of *noise* when it comes to the topic of slenderizing our bodies—and the volume gets louder once you're expecting a baby and then adjusting to life as a new mom.

After more than a decade of work as beauty activists, we came to a profound realization: Pregnancy and new motherhood are the times when women go through the most insecurity-inducing body changes and when we have the *least* support to deal with those changes. By *support* we don't mean the onslaught of articles that reveal which new mom celebrities fit back in their bikinis in five minutes by "just eating healthy," or the "mommy makeover" specials that are increasingly prevalent on plastic surgeons' Web sites. Neither of these are on our list of self-esteem boosters.

At the other end of the spectrum are the Bad Mommy Police, who will make women feel incredibly selfish for giving a minute's thought to how we look when we should be showering every ounce of our attention onto our new bundles of joy. Don't worry: There is a middle ground—and we will help you find yours, if you are pregnant, considering getting pregnant, or are home with baby.

We first met when Claire was the director of an eating disorders organization, a position she took after finally giving up her dangerous quest to be model-thin. Magali was an internationally renowned model who wanted to reveal the truths she knew about the fashion industry—the rampant retouching, the insane pressures on insanely young models, the difference between the pretty fantasies on those glossy magazine covers and the ugly realities of her real-life eating disorder. We teamed up with the goal of educating and raising awareness. However, as we traveled around the country talking to women, we quickly learned that the main event was not the stories we were sharing, but the stories other women shared with us. Concerned women would fling their hands up in the air and ask what they could say to their friends who weren't eating enough. Others lined up to tell us how exasperated they felt after years of yo-yo dieting, or to share their secret behavior that "wasn't an eating disorder" but something else—something they hadn't confessed to anyone until that day. We saw the shame as women hesitated, and then continued with their stories. We recognized that shame because we'd felt it ourselves.

Magali got pregnant in 2005 and Claire got married in 2006. Motherhood was no longer some distant role we might someday step into, but something very real. We talked about how strange it was to suddenly find the details of Magali's pregnancy weight gain an acceptable topic of daily discussion at business lunches

A Silent Majority

Seventy-eight percent of women we surveyed who do not have children yet or do not plan to have children told us they have concerns about how pregnancy and motherhood could change their bodies. Most of them keep those concerns to themselves. Fifty-seven percent said they don't talk about the connections among pregnancy, motherhood, and body image with their friends. Fifty-one percent said they never discuss it with their partners.

and among friends, especially after all the years she'd invested in shifting her focus *away* from that number on the scale. We took notice of what other pregnant women and new mothers were talking about—and what they weren't. There was plenty of chatter about how everyone wanted to lose their baby weight and not lose themselves in motherhood, but how were women really coping with those pressures? There were shelves filled with books about work-life balance and op-ed pages devoted to "mommy wars" and "opting out." Where was the thoughtful exploration of how pregnancy and motherhood changes a woman's relationship to her body and her sense of beauty and style? Tabloid baby bump-watch covers just weren't cutting it for us.

We asked real women—over four hundred of them—about their biggest body concerns related to pregnancy and motherhood. We heard from first-time mothers, veteran moms, women who don't have children yet, and pregnant women who described themselves as everything from "sexy" to "heffalump." We also managed to track down some husbands and partners who were willing to give us the scoop on what they think about the expanding bellies, raging hormones, and what sex is like after baby arrives.

The women we interviewed made us crack up, cry, and believe with ever more conviction that when we women are honest with ourselves and with each other, we are unstoppable.

We want women to feel less alone. We want mothers and mothers-to-be to know that worrying about your appearance doesn't make you selfish or unfit for parenting. It's what you choose to *do* about those concerns that matters the most. For us, staying silent and waiting to see what happens are never options. We're also not fans of the everything-will-be-okay-as-long-as-I-can-get-back-into-my-skinny-jeans approach. So while we will not be offering the secrets to getting your prebaby body back, this book *will* serve up some practical tips on how to love and respect your body through the amazing, awe-inspiring, and, yes, sometimes downright shocking changes of pregnancy and motherhood. We'll tell you all about those changes and you'll hear from women who have lived through them. We will provide real-life solutions for women who care about their looks *and* their babies, but are not going to be working out for two hours a day anytime soon (or ever). We'll offer advice for those who have struggled to accept their bodies, only to face the absolute certainty of weight gain in pregnancy and the complete uncertainty of how they'll cope with it. We'll give you the uncensored truth about everything from milky boobs to prebaby bikini waxes. Celebrities, style, beauty, fitness, and body-image experts will all weigh in; and we'll throw our two cents into the mix as well.

From the "What am I getting myself into?" side of things is Claire, who has a major case of baby fever and plans to do something about it soon. In the "been there, survived that" category is Magali, who is understanding more and more each day how the reflection she sees of herself shapes the reflection her daughter sees when she looks in the mirror.

We won't sugarcoat this for you. The stakes are much higher when you bring kids into the picture. Of course, you won't always feel like a beautiful, glowing goddess—and that's okay. But even after one of those "ugly" days, every woman deserves to go to sleep believing deeply and implicitly in her own beauty. Our children need us to believe in our beauty. Each morning you wake up feeling stronger and more confident, you will be better prepared to help your daughters and sons find *their* strength and confidence.

1

Body Basics: Pregnancy and Beyond

Get healthy before you get pregnant. It's a noble and sensible goal, but what are we really talking about when we talk about health? Is it something you can claim when you reach a certain number on the scale? Is it the specific tally of hours and minutes you spend at the gym each week, or the calories or fat grams you consume? Many of us slam into a confounding roadblock when we try to prepare for motherhood: We've spent our lives struggling to accept our bodies, trying to lose weight or diet down to the size we think will make us happy, but we've never experienced what it feels like to be healthy with no numbers attached. We sometimes feel inadequate, unpretty, inferior. On the one hand, we're anxious about how our bodies will change during pregnancy and what we will look like as mothers. On the other hand, we are terrified of passing those fears and insecurities on to our children.

Weight and size are central to so many women's thoughts and conversations: I weigh X. I need to lose X pounds. I just bought a dress in a size X! But when it comes to starting a family, we need to start thinking about *health* in broader terms: I love X form of exercise. I eat X amount of fruits and vegetables. I know X is an issue that makes me feel insecure about my body or eat in unhealthy ways. Dieting and weight preoccupation will not get us ready for motherhood—self-reflection and body confidence will.

Body image: The internal picture of how you see your outward appearance, which doesn't always match what others see. Have you ever dismissed someone who says you look beautiful because what you see in the mirror looks ugly? The self-portrait you carry with you profoundly affects how you feel and how you interact with others in the world. And it's a two-way street, because how you feel and how you interact can shape the way you see yourself.

Body confidence: The belief that you are your most beautiful when you are healthy—both in body and mind. A feeling that results when you give up the mission to mold and shape yourself and make the commitment to take care of yourself. Body confidence breeds positive body image— it enables us to see ourselves through a meaningful lens, not a superficial one.

How We See Ourselves

"I do have a poor body image. Not a lot of people know because I act very confident, but I am constantly comparing myself to others. I am sure that 90 percent of women feel the same way I do." —Shannon, 25

"Is there a woman in America who does not have a poor body image? It has nothing to do with what you look like, whether you're thin or not. You can still have issues." —Walkiria, 39

"Well, what girl doesn't have a poor body image? I've always wanted to be skinnier than I am." —Nicole, 24

"Fixating on my body in an unhealthy way, scrutinizing food choices, etc., was quite 'normal' within my social circle, so it never seemed like a problem until I started to learn about these issues and think more about body image in our society." —Sabrina, 22

Before, During, and After: Women's Top Fears

Women were crystal clear when we asked them what pregnancy and mommy-related body changes they were most concerned about. As Maria, forty years old and thirty-one weeks pregnant put it succinctly, "Duh. Not being able to lose the weight." Women who don't have children yet are nervous about gaining pregnancy weight and losing it after the baby is born. Expectant moms want to gain exactly the right amount of weight during pregnancy and lose it quickly after the baby is born. And new mothers are eager to . . . wouldn't you know it? Lose weight.

It's not just that women are vaguely concerned about weight. In some cases, they are downright terrified. "I don't want to be the big, fat, gross behemoth mom in sweatpants," says Heather, thirty-six, and in her twentieth week of pregnancy. "Will I end up with a ruined body?" echoes Lila, forty-one. Even those who discuss body fears other than weight are prone to hyperbole. "I'm afraid my boobs will hang down to the floor," says Ellen, twenty-three.

The legend of Saggy-Boobed Behemoth Mom lives mostly in the imaginations of women who believe that pregnancy and motherhood will upset the delicate balance they've worked so hard to achieve—and that the forty weeks off their typical diet and workout plan will unleash an insatiable beast. "I'm afraid the way I keep thin now (calorie counting, exercising daily) would no longer work," says Michelle, twenty-eight.

Ultimately, women worry that this loss of control will cause them to lose a grip on who they are. "I realize that I can't know how any of this will play out until I am actually in the midst of it," admits Amy, twenty-five. "I imagine that once I am pregnant and

Weighty Fears

Seventy-nine percent of the women who have body fears related to motherhood name *weight* (getting bigger during pregnancy and not being able to lose the weight after delivery) as their number-one fear.

then a new mother, I would have plenty of concerns other than how I look or how my body looks. That in and of itself freaks me out a bit because I have always been thin/fit/healthy and I feel that is part of my identity and a priority." Sonja, thirty-one, says she is also thinking more about the connection between her body image and her identity. "I worry that my body will change so significantly that I will no longer feel like myself."

Your Top Body Fears: Uncensored

While weight is overwhelmingly women's top concern, there are a few other body fears that make the list:

✓ Stretch Marks
✓ Sagging Breasts, Bigger Breasts, Deflated Breasts, Darker Nipples
✓ Flabby Stomach, Huge Belly, Stretched Navel
✓ Loose Vagina
✓ Swollen Feet
✓ Wider Hips
✓ Hemorrhoids
✓ Varicose Veins
✓ Incontinence
✓ Skin Trouble
✓ Hair Falling Out
✓ Episiotomy

Will you have to deal with everything on that list? It's unlikely. But we'll be honest: Those fears aren't based on fiction. Frankly, some of them can be a real pain in the ass (and in the case of one item, we mean that literally). We are here to help you face whatever you have to go through so you can come out the other side with your self-esteem intact. The first thing you need to know is that plenty of real women—and their partners—have managed to survive all sorts of body changes that came along with pregnancy and new motherhood.

The Real Deal

On breasts: *"I got* National Geographic *nipples!"*   —Jennifer, 40

On the postbaby vagina (a guy's perspective): *"I remember the first time I slept with a woman who had given birth. That was when I discovered that women who had children knew their vaginal muscles a lot better than those with no kids."*   —Yannis, 35

On stretch marks: *"I was very worried about stretch marks and used cocoa butter daily after showering [see "The Miracle Stretch-Mark Cream," page 112], but only on my stomach. I had no idea that I would get them anywhere else and wound up getting them on my butt."* —Jen, 37

"I seriously thought I'd be forced to start a bold/bald model trend after giving birth to my daughter. But other than the roadkill-looking clumps I would find on my pillow in the morning and the clogged drain in my shower, there were no other obvious signs that I was shedding. No one else noticed and after a few months, things went back to normal."   —Magali, on her experience with hair loss

Body Confidence 101:
When You're Planning a Family

While many women tell us they want to lose weight before they get pregnant, only rarely do they talk about trying to make peace with their bodies. They are quick to share dieting triumphs and failures, but they don't mention anything about getting in touch with their natural appetites or figuring out the reasons *why* they overeat, restrict their caloric intake, or yo-yo. "Most of my girlfriends want children—even though they are obsessed with their weight," says Michelle, twenty-eight. "I don't understand how they expect to have all these children and remain a size 0." Contrary to popular belief, emotional and physical health are not automatic prizes handed to us when we reach some "ideal" weight. There are thin women who hate their bodies and have screwed-up relationships with food, and there are fat women who are healthy, active, and confident in who they are. As you prepare to become a mother, take the scale out of the equation for long enough to ask yourself these two questions:

1. What attitudes about food, weight, and body image do you want to instill in your child?

2. Do those attitudes match your own?

We're not arguing that you have to be the model of perfect body image before you decide to start a family. In fact, we'd like every woman to wipe that word *perfect* out of her vocabulary right now. You might still have those days when nothing in your closet looks good when you try it on. You might still be tempted to denigrate yourself to others. You don't have to have it all figured out. But what are you doing to work toward body *confidence*? Are you digging deep to address the reasons why you don't like what you see when you look in the mirror?

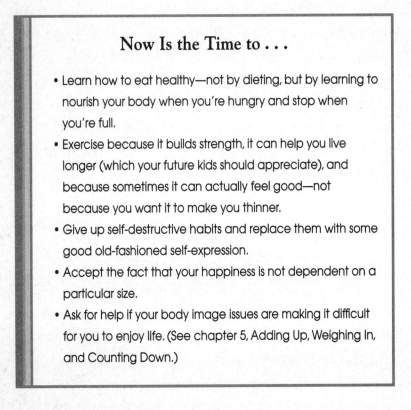

Now Is the Time to . . .

- Learn how to eat healthy—not by dieting, but by learning to nourish your body when you're hungry and stop when you're full.
- Exercise because it builds strength, it can help you live longer (which your future kids should appreciate), and because sometimes it can actually feel good—not because you want it to make you thinner.
- Give up self-destructive habits and replace them with some good old-fashioned self-expression.
- Accept the fact that your happiness is not dependent on a particular size.
- Ask for help if your body image issues are making it difficult for you to enjoy life. (See chapter 5, Adding Up, Weighing In, and Counting Down.)

Claire says:

"My body already is, and has always been, changing. I don't have the same body today as I did in my twenties. I didn't have the same body in my twenties as I did in my teens. And there were some pretty noticeable changes happening from birth to adolescence, too. Sure, pregnancy and motherhood bring a whole new world of changes in a short amount of time, and that's scary for anyone who has a history of body issues—me included. But I know I don't want to waste any of my precious energy trying to fight change. I've done enough battle with my body. We called a truce."

Your doctor will tell you it's best to develop healthy habits before you start a family. Reflect on what that really means, because the state of your health is not just about how much you weigh; it's about how you approach food, exercise, and your emotions. How healthy you are is a result of how you cope with stress, how you express your feelings, and how much—or how little—body confidence you have.

Body Confidence 101: While You're Pregnant

Anyone and everyone can tell you that your body will go through some major transformations while you're pregnant. No one can tell you exactly how you will feel about those changes and what pregnancy will be like for you. Some women love every minute of it, while others are counting the minutes until it's over. There might be days when you can't imagine anything better and days when you doubt there could be anything worse. The point is that there is no "right" way to experience pregnancy. You're not required to be over-the-moon happy all the time. In fact, pretending everything's peachy when you feel all-around crappy can be a real confidence killer.

"I would rather be dangling on a one-hundred-foot pole by my feet than be pregnant," says Kristen, thirty-four. While she hated her two pregnancies from beginning to end, what made them even tougher was that she felt like she couldn't open up about how miserable she was. "I wish more people had been more honest about their pregnancies to say when they had a hard time, too. My friends would not understand. They would say, 'You are so lucky! You're pregnant, you have a great husband, what are you complaining about?' I would have to respect that. I know that at my age, women come from a lot of different experiences of trying to get pregnant or married."

To Each Her Own

"It was the happiest I had been in my life. I was content with myself. It was an incredibly comfortable pregnancy. The kicking and moving inside of me was intensely calming." —Stephanie, 26

"Pregnancy sucks. It's awful. Not awful for everyone, but it certainly was for me. It is worth it, I must say. I do think motherhood is certainly the most gratifying thing I've done in my life." —Debbie, 38

"I felt very beautiful, sexy, and kind of invincible." —Taiia, 35

"I think one of the myths out there is that pregnant women are so happy. Really? I kind of feel like shit and I'm tired of going to the bathroom every eight minutes. Then you almost feel guilty about that and you start asking yourself, 'Should I be embracing this pregnancy?' I think some people do feel really great, but some of us don't, and that's okay." —Amy, 37

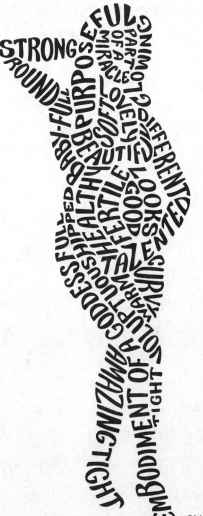

©Monica Martinez

We asked women to describe their pregnant bodies. There was little hesitation—the words came flooding our way in a stream of extremes.

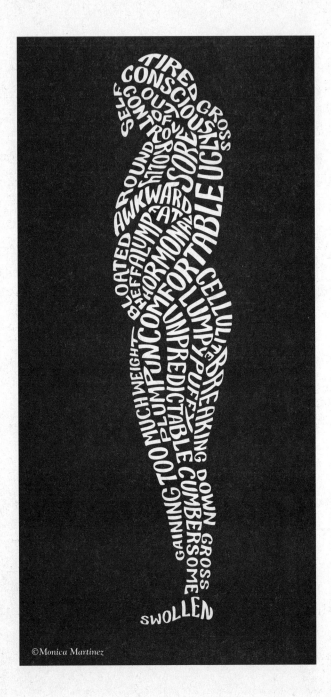

©Monica Martinez

Body confidence comes from believing that beauty is connected to your physical and emotional health. So if you're constipated, exhausted, swollen, nauseated, or dealing with any number of other pregnancy-related ailments, it's no wonder you don't feel gorgeous! All we ask is that you not keep those frustrations to yourself because you're afraid to let on that you are not the picture of the blissful, glowing pregnancy. You might be hesitant to call up your girlfriends to moan about your hemorrhoids, but you should at least call your doctor and ask what you can do to get some relief. And if the stress of weight gain, loss of control, or other changes in your body are causing you to suffer, reach out. Ask for support to deal with whatever issues and fears are making you unhappy. Yes, there are some out there who will deem your worries "silly." Forget about them. You owe it yourself and your child to find the people who won't dismiss your concerns. Take care of your body and your mind. If there's one thing we've learned, it's that silence is not good for either.

In Her Own Words:

When Your Pregnancy Is Far from Perfect

When I got pregnant, I had been working on my doctoral dissertation and working as an instructor at a community college. When I went into preterm labor and was put on bed rest, the doctor wouldn't allow me to sit up at the computer, and the medicine they gave me to control the contractions made it hard to concentrate anyway, so I couldn't work on my dissertation.

Actually, this was very liberating for me, as I had not allowed myself to read novels for all the years that I had been studying, so I really enjoyed reading novels. I did feel isolated and lonely because we had just moved to the area and I didn't really know anyone, and all of our family lived out of state. I think that having people visit would have helped and I would recommend to other women in that situation that they try and arrange to have other people visit. If nothing else, it would be a distraction. I recall feeling bad because I knew other women who were pregnant at the same time and weren't having any complications at all. I did learn to appreciate not moving and remaining calm (my daughter was a very calm baby/child and I wonder if my bed rest didn't influence that in some way). I also focused on one day at a time. If you look at the time all at once, it is devastating, but only focusing on one day at a time is not so bad. I also think that I had imagined being pregnant and enjoying it long before I was pregnant, and it was hard to realize that my "dream pregnancy" was not going to occur. Likewise, the increased and ever-present anxiety that at any moment I could lose the pregnancy was difficult. Again, I chose to not think about it by putting myself in the fantasy of fiction (while reading) most of the time.

Even though I basically had the pregnancy from hell, once born, my baby was 100 percent healthy and beautiful, she was calm and cheerful, and is a very smart and, more important, a very good person at 13 years old today—so a bad pregnancy doesn't mean that your baby will have problems later on.

Cheryl, 50

Where's My Cute Baby Bump?

Pregnancy is a big waiting game. There are milestones and markers—and more milestones and markers. For many women, the one they can't wait to reach (besides the baby's arrival, of course) is the point when they actually start to look pregnant.

"For the first three months, I couldn't feel the baby. There was nothing solid telling me I was changing for a reason, so I started to feel uncomfortable about the way I looked because I did start to gain weight and there was no legitimate reason in my mind for the weight gain," remembers Mary, thirty-one.

Lisa, thirty-five, also had a hard time with the idea that her belly wasn't the only part of her that was getting rounder. "When I started gaining weight, it was really disheartening because at first it was only in my hips and thighs," she remembers. "I thought, 'Well, wait a second, where's my cute little baby bump?' No, I'm gaining weight in my hips and thighs. The baby's not in there, so why am I gaining all this weight? Before I was pregnant, when I would see a pregnant woman, I would say, 'Who cares how much weight you're gaining? You're creating a life. You're a goddess! Who cares?' And then when it's you . . .'"

No matter how excited you are about your pregnancy, that initial weight gain can be a shock if you have body insecurities. That's one of the reasons why we recommend some preemptive closet cleaning (see New Addition, New You: Style & Beauty for Expectant and New Moms, page 89), which will help you avoid the frustration of discovering that you are too big to squeeze into your favorite pencil skirt when you don't yet have a pregnant belly to offer the world as an obvious explanation for your expansion.

At the first sign that your body is getting bigger, remind yourself that this is what is *supposed* to be happening. Women tend to waste a lot of energy worrying about whether we're doing things the way we "should" be doing them. Pregnancy can kick that impulse into overdrive. And it's not only that we want to do everything just right; there's the added pressure of looking just right, too. But if you start wishing for the "perfect" (there's that nasty word again!) pregnant body from the outset, you are bound to be disappointed. Pregnancies are like snowflakes—albeit oversized snowflakes that don't exactly float through the air. The point is that no two look exactly alike, and none is inherently more beautiful than another.

"I remember clearly the day I saw a picture online of Salma Hayek looking huge," says Erica, thirty-eight. "To me, that was reassuring. She was not a little bump. She was a big woman with big breasts and a big belly. That was an image and a role model for me—a big, very pregnant woman. And she looked totally great!"

Your body will work some serious magic in the coming months. Wherever and whenever you find that extra padding, keep in mind that it's all part of this package called pregnancy.

Eating for Two

Dieting is pretty much a national pastime. Every day, millions of women are counting calories, cutting carbs, declaring certain foods "off-limits," and feeling guilty when they can't achieve the results they want through all that restriction and deprivation. It's not surprising that many of them are quick to highlight what they loved most about pregnancy: the freedom to eat and to get bigger.

"My favorite part was eating everything I wanted to!" recalls Angela, thirty-six. And this permission to eat can also come with a reprieve from the usual body hatred we subject ourselves to. "I felt good about my body in a way I never do otherwise. I felt sexy and proud and pretty most of the time because I felt like I had an 'excuse' to have a giant stomach," says Jenni, thirty-eight.

The only problem with this "pregnancy as a vacation" concept is that it's temporary. If you believe pregnancy is the only time in your life when you are allowed to eat without guilt and accept the size of your body, what happens when the pregnancy party is over? Get ready for one harsh comedown.

In many cases, women gain more pregnancy weight than they needed to because a lifetime of dieting screws up their ability to trust their natural appetites. That can lead to poor eating habits and sometimes even bingeing (see chapter 5, Adding Up, Weighing In, and Counting Down, for more on bingeing during pregnancy) if they abandon a lifetime's worth of strict, self-imposed rules related to eating.

Our solution is pretty basic. *Stop dieting*—not just during pregnancy, but before and after pregnancy, too. If that one stopped you in your tracks, we hope you'll hear us out. We're calling B.S. on the pregnancy free pass because we believe the freedom to eat and not be ashamed of your body isn't just a treat that comes with being pregnant; it's a freedom women should have *every day*. Dieting strips us of that freedom. The more you diet, the more difficult it is to know when you are truly hungry and when to stop when you're satisfied. We want women to learn how to nourish their bodies and exercise for their health instead of obsessing about reaching a goal weight.

Diets Don't Work

A comprehensive review of 31 long-term diet studies, published in the April 2007 issue of *American Psychologist* and conducted by researchers at UCLA, revealed that the majority of people who lost weight on diets will gain it back, and then some. The authors of the study concluded that dieting is actually a consistent predictor of future weight *gain*.

If you were dieting before your pregnancy, consider this an opportunity to reset your system, grow a healthy baby, and work on being the healthiest mom you can be. You might need some extra help to overcome the all-or-nothing mind-set that can result from going on and off diets. A nutritionist can give you guidance on making smart food choices now and in the future. A counselor can work with you to understand the roots of your past weight struggles and move you closer to the healthy place you want to be as a mother. Those resources are out there for you. Don't be afraid to use them.

Information Overload!

The amount of conflicting information about what you should or shouldn't do, eat, drink, think about, breathe, use, look at, or touch while pregnant is enough to drive you nuts. And speaking of nuts . . . One study we found says you can eat all the peanuts you want. But wait! Absolutely no peanuts allowed, according to another study. If you want to know that it's okay to drink coffee or alcohol in moderation, we've got research to back up that argument. And we've got studies and experts to say they are both no-no's, too. Where is the truth in all this? Well, it comes down to you, your doctor, and your intuition. Trust yourself and your body. We know pregnancy can make you a little loopy, but it doesn't wipe out your basic common sense.

Magali says:

"I grew up in France, where wine flows freely and pregnant women are not given the death stare for having an occasional drink. I had decided that I would go with that approach during my pregnancy, but my body told me otherwise. I just had no desire for wine during those months. It wasn't a big deal or a huge decision to make—I just went with what felt right for me."

The New Numbers Game

We both threw away our scales long ago. Our focus on numbers was keeping us trapped in comparisons and self-criticism. The fluctuations of pounds held way too much power over us, so we trashed those scales and rebooted our lives without them. After a while, we stopped wondering about where that needle might land and we learned how to eat and exercise without the looming fear or hopeful anticipation of what the scale would have to say about it. We let our doctors weigh us, but with the understanding that we didn't want to know the number unless it was specifically related to a health concern.

This plan was working out just swimmingly—until Magali got pregnant. That is when she discovered (and was kind enough to give Claire the heads-up) that avoiding the topic of weight during pregnancy is like steering clear of sand on a beach. However, while it might be impossible to control the fact that people will constantly ask you about your weight, tell you how much weight they gained during pregnancy, and how they lost it afterwards, you can still take *your* number out of the mix. Or better yet, replace it with a new one.

Magali says:

"My weight had been a trigger for unhealthy thoughts and behavior (see chapter 5, Adding Up, Weighing In, and Counting Down), so I had no interest in knowing or discussing how much I weighed throughout my pregnancy. But I did find a fun way to record the radical physical changes my body was going through: I measured my belly length—from my back to the end of my popped-out belly button. I am usually not fond of numbers, but I will gladly disclose that one. I was two feet wide! Every time I think of it, it makes me smile."

You don't have to get rid of your scale if you don't think an awareness of your weight will bother you. But be mindful of the fact that pregnancy is a time when many other people will be keenly interested in that number, too. Those conversations can be a trip . . . and not always a good one (see chapter 7, The WTF Files: How to Deal with Dumb Comments and Stupid Moves). Pregnancy should be a time to concentrate on taking care of your body and your baby. Numbers can sometimes distract us from that very important task.

There Really Is a Baby in There!

The sensation of your baby moving inside you can be incredibly powerful, inspiring, and maybe even a little scary. For many mothers-to-be, that first kick can also kick-start a new appreciation of their bodies that isn't based on size or weight.

"I loved watching my belly grow and feeling life move around inside me. It's amazing what your body is capable of."   —Amanda, 30

"I was in awe of my changing body. It actually helped me respect my body in a whole new light."   —Marina, 31

"There was an energy that I felt most days—it was the same energy I think people saw when they said that I was glowing. It's hard to

describe and it's different for everyone, but embrace the power and energy you can feel when you're pregnant. I think some women miss that feeling because they focus too much on the weight gain."

—Veronica, 33

"The closeness I felt to the little McFetus was really great, and also something that was all mine." —Mara, 35

Keep It Moving

You can't have body confidence if you don't move your body. Exercise should be a regular part of your life. That goes for during pregnancy, too—unless you have been instructed to avoid certain activities. Talk to your doctor about what types and amounts of exercise are safe for your pregnancy and don't push yourself too hard or try anything new and strenuous.

Mary Powell owns LillySerpentine Fusion Bellydance in Bozeman, Montana. She first started belly dancing after a friend dragged her to a class and was instantly hooked by the sense of community she witnessed. "I was enthralled with the dancing. It was just all shapes and sizes of women from different backgrounds. Really, belly dancing is a way for women to get together and feel confident in themselves. We can talk about the uncomfortable parts of our bodies and dance it out."

Mary continued belly dancing during her pregnancy and found that it kept her connected to everything that was going on with her body, which makes a lot of sense because belly dancing was actually used as a ritual to prepare women for birth in ancient times.

"I danced twice a week throughout the whole pregnancy and

taught classes. There were so many emotions—it was wonderful," she remembers. "I performed a month before I was due with my big belly showing and everything. I could feel every movement. Even in the pictures you could see where the baby was lying. I was glowing inside and out."

Exercise comes in many forms. What's most important is that you find movement that feels good and helps you build strength during your pregnancy.

Claire says:

"I take walks around my neighborhood and I've started noticing this pregnant woman who must be on the same walking schedule. I can really feel her power when we pass each other. She's moving fast, arms pumping, and just *owning* the space around her. I am now officially her secret cheerleader."

Magali says:

"I am a yoga fan. I am biased, because my mother's a teacher. During my pregnancy I continued my regular classes. I tried prenatal yoga, and even though I enjoyed being in a room filled with expecting moms, it wasn't for me. In my third trimester, when I started getting physically uncomfortable, I tried swimming. It rocked my pregnant world! Gravity relief was all the balance I needed to have more energy during my day. I absolutely loved it, looked forward to it, and made friends with all the elderly YMCA swimmers who became my afternoon companions. My body was able to relax and remain strong—all the while thoroughly delighting in the sensation of the water on my belly as I pictured my daughter 'swimming' simultaneously in her own mama-made pool!"

Can You Plan for Birth?

There is an endgame to pregnancy. It's this thing called birth. When you imagine what it will be like to meet your little one for the first time, what do you picture? Do you see yourself in a particular place? Who are the people surrounding you? Are you comfortably numb or are you going for it au naturel? These are some of the key questions you need to ask yourself and discuss with your health care provider. Gather information, decide what would be best for you, and make what we prefer to call your birth "wish list." Because the truth is that when Junior arrives, there is every possibility that your plans might take a flying leap out the window.

"It's not a practical thing and this is where I get angry. You pick up any pregnancy book and it will have a whole thing about the birth plan," Hermione, forty-four, exclaimed when we asked her about her thoughts on the idea of a birth plan. "I'll tell you what the birth plan is—it's an oxy-fucking-moron! There is no such thing as a plan for birth."

Patience, Intuition, and a Handbag

"I definitely had ideas in my head and the mind-set to have the baby naturally. I wanted to have the baby in the birth center and I was going to be hanging out in the Jacuzzi. We would make soup to take with us. Somebody was going to bake cookies. There was this sense that it was going to be a really big celebration with all my friends and family around me. As it turned out, I was in the hospital lots of hours, I did have an epidural, I couldn't get out of bed, and I couldn't move.

It was very, very different from what I had planned. I definitely felt like my body had failed me. It's hard, but you have to be patient with yourself and forgiving of yourself. Set your plan but don't set it in stone, because it will never be exactly the way you plan it." —Jen, 32

"I think it's important to maintain your intuition and that sense of your own body through pregnancy, birth, and afterwards. If you feel that something is going wrong, then something is going wrong. But if you feel like everything is going right and you're being pressured into something you don't want to do, don't rush into it. Take a breath and ask yourself: How are you feeling? Are you ready for what is being proposed? When giving birth, I had a very long labor. They offered me a C-section. I know myself and I know myself physically. I knew I had a strong baby. I had her inside me and I knew that she could make it out." —Natalia, 35

"Someone told me beforehand that having a C-section feels like someone rummaging around in a handbag, only the handbag is your abdomen. It repulsed me when I first heard it, but it seemed funny during the surgery because that's exactly what it feels like! Our daughter was delivered, warmed up, and handed to my husband while the surgeons sewed me up. My husband brought the baby over to me and I held her and looked into her eyes, but she couldn't breast-feed right away because of the meds in my bloodstream. We cuddled more in the recovery room and worked on breastfeeding over the following few days." —Sandra, 38

You should absolutely educate yourself about the birth process and take steps to lay the groundwork for the kind of delivery you want to have. But you should also recognize that things don't always go according to plan. "You can't go into birth with a script and expect that it's going to go that way because you just don't know. Things can happen and you have to be flexible," advises Sherry Rumsey, a certified doula. "The big keys are to educate yourself and to be with a care provider and support people you trust. If a woman is educated going in, and she knows her options and knows what different things to try, she can say, 'I know I did what I could.' That's not to say that she won't feel some loss if things go differently than she wanted. But it's easier to face it, get past it, and move on to mothering."

It doesn't hurt to have a picture of your ideal birth in your mind. Just remind yourself that you will make the decisions that feel right and your body will do its job. You have to make room for the many possibilities of how that job might get done.

Body Confidence 101: After Delivery

You will be flooded with all kinds of emotions (not to mention a megadose of hormones) after you give birth. If you are a first-time mom, you will probably be staring into the eyes of a tiny newborn while trying to wrap your brain around your new title: MOTHER. You might also be frantically opening and closing the drawers of your nightstand looking for the take-home *Mommy Manual* they surely must have given you at the hospital. They can't really expect you to know what to do with this little person once you're on your own with no nurse on call!

Welcome to the next stage in your life. Whether things went exactly as planned or they strayed far from the course you had imagined, what is most important is that you and your baby made it to this moment. Your body brought this child into the world. And here you are.

Magali says:

"I remember my first shower in my own bathroom after I came home from the hospital with my daughter. I looked down at my body in awe. For the first time, I saw it as an incredible machine, and I realized what an astoundingly complex mystery it was to me. I thought of all those years of abuse I had put it through and how resilient it had been. What my body had accomplished was a miracle and I was proud of it. I said, 'Thank you' out loud."

Many of us have found ourselves in adversarial relationships with our bodies throughout our lives. We want thinner legs or firmer stomachs. We want to take some curves from here and put them there. We're quick to zero in on the parts we wish were different. But birth requires us to work—and by work, we mean *labor*—with what we've got. Before you get stymied by stretch marks and fixated on flabby skin, remember to take a look at your baby and take pride in your body. Yes, you did that!

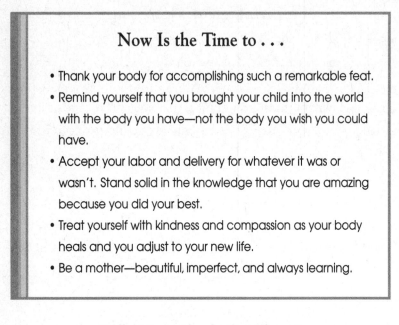

Now Is the Time to . . .

- Thank your body for accomplishing such a remarkable feat.
- Remind yourself that you brought your child into the world with the body you have—not the body you wish you could have.
- Accept your labor and delivery for whatever it was or wasn't. Stand solid in the knowledge that you are amazing because you did your best.
- Treat yourself with kindness and compassion as your body heals and you adjust to your new life.
- Be a mother—beautiful, imperfect, and always learning.

Hello? Is Anybody Out There?

Remember all those regular doctor's appointments you had throughout your pregnancy? There were tests and measurements and check-ins galore to make sure that everything was progressing properly. You developed a relationship with your health care provider as your baby grew. Hopefully, if it was a good relationship, you felt that someone was looking out for you. But your doctor or midwife's big job is done after delivery (in this country, at least), which means that many women come home from the hospital or the birthing center to the proverbial sound of crickets chirping and the actual sound of a screaming newborn. Most obstetricians and midwives will schedule a check-in for six weeks after your delivery. "A lot of things can happen in six weeks. And a lot of women are not going to rush back to their OB. They feel like that relationship is basically over, so there's this gap in maternity care in that postpartum period. They have the pediatrician for the baby, but who do the moms see?" asks Sherry Rumsey, a doula who does in-home postpartum visits with new mothers two weeks after they give birth.

Whether or not you hire a doula, be aware that it's not just your baby's health you should be tending to after you give birth; your health is important, too. In fact, if you are in a significant amount of physical or emotional pain, it will be very hard for you to mother your new baby. Pick up the phone and call your doctor as soon as you have a question, if you feel depressed, or you need more options for pain relief. You don't have to wait six weeks.

Is This More Than the Baby Blues?

It is very common to experience mood swings, weepy episodes, and feelings of being overwhelmed in the days after you give birth. Whatever it is you're going through, express yourself and make sure your partner or at least one person you trust knows how you are feeling. In most cases your hormones will level out and you'll start feeling more stable and ready to deal. But if you can't shake the darkness, reach out.

"What I tell women in the hospital is that postpartum depression doesn't feel like you want to put your baby in the oven or throw your baby out the window. That's postpartum psychosis and that is very rare. Depression can feel like your mind won't rest, and what you're anxious about are things that are probably not worth obsessing about. Even when the lights are out and the baby is sleeping, you are obsessing. Sometimes you have irrational but scary thoughts," notes Christina Adberg, M.D., an OB/GYN. "Once in a while, I get a call from someone three months post-partum and she'll say, 'I don't have postpartum depression, but I think I'm just really anxious.' I try to get women to open up earlier. But it is better for them to be treated later than not at all. Oftentimes, women don't accept it and they don't want to be the one who has it."

Don't work yourself up into a frenzy worrying about whether you will develop postpartum depression. Educate yourself about the signs, symptoms, and risk factors (women with a history of depression and eating disorders have a higher risk of developing postpartum depression), and keep your support system close at hand. Postpartum depression can be treated. Make a commitment to yourself that you will reach out if you need help.

Your New Body: What Really Happens After Delivery

There are plenty of red carpet "postbaby body" debuts mere weeks after celebrities give birth (see chapter 2, "Media Madness"), but we don't see a lot of new moms' bodies in the real world—mainly because most new moms are recovering at home, trying to juggle poopy diapers, feedings, pain, sleep, and the decoding of various baby-screaming pitches—all in a semi zombified state. "It's not like in the commercials. It's not all easy. You need to adjust to the new situation. Your body healing takes time. But it gets easier every day. Don't worry—you're a good mom. Take your time," says Cat, thirty-six.

New Mom Body Confessions

"A lot of women probably don't like all that wobbly loose flesh, but I actually liked it. I found it to be like a souvenir or proof of this really wonderful thing that had happened. I was really elated and I would lift my T-shirt and be like, 'Look at all this! It's brilliant!' *And that's not like me to behave like that."*   —Sarah, 32

"I had the worst flatulence of my life after giving birth. It would smell like somebody died in our room. And nobody tells you about that! And the bleeding. And the night sweats and the dripping milk and the hemorrhoids. That was really, really gross."   —Mara, 35

"I don't really know if I'm the same shape and size down there. I kept asking, 'Is this normal? Is this normal?' And my midwife said to me, 'It might be your new normal.'"   —Diane, 34

"I try to be proud of my stretch marks. They are scars worth being proud of, but they were also a shock."   —Sara, 31

"Your body changes shape and you have to come to terms with it. I now weigh less than I did before the pregnancy, but I am still bigger in most places of concern (stomach and chest). My body is just not the same shape as it was. I notice myself in the mirror every once in a while and it jolts me a little, but I don't think about it all that much."

—Anna, 35

Listen up, new moms. Your body just went through something major. You are resilient and powerful, but you are not a rubber band. Your belly might very well resemble a Jell-O mold right now;

that doesn't mean it will look that way forever. However, you do have to get used to the fact that some things about your body *are* permanently changed, and those changes can be the toughest to accept, especially when so many magazines and mommy groups are filled with chatter about how to get your body back. Unless you want to erase the newest addition to your family and all the hard work you did to nurture that little baby to life, you need to make a conscious decision that you are not going to set body goals for yourself that involve stepping into a time machine.

Body Talk: The Conversations That Matter

Accepting your new body is not as simple as flipping on the Confident Mommy switch. Moments of insecurity are inevitable, so don't pile on more guilt and pressure when you have them. "You want to think it's totally okay to look however you want to look, but that's not the world we live in," admits Amy, thirty-seven. "I've learned to tell myself that it's okay to care about these things. I think that's the catch-22 with women. You feel bad about your body, and then you feel bad that you feel bad about it. I should be stronger and more confident than that! On an intellectual level, I look at my friends and I don't care what they look like. But I care what I look like."

One of the best ways we can work toward body confidence is to talk about our issues. The problem is that women have absolutely no idea how to have these conversations with each other. Either we are tiptoeing around the glaring problems or we are spinning our wheels in completely unhelpful conversations filled with meaningless reassurances and comparisons. It's not our fault—we never learned how to speak any other language. We all need a Vocab Rehab.

Vocab Rehab

Scene 1:

"God, you should have told me my ass looks enormous in these jeans," a woman exclaims to her girlfriend after catching her profile in a store window.

"Oh, please. You look great. It's my ham-size upper arms we should be talking about," the friend responds.

Vocab Rehab . . .

"God, you should have told me my ass looks enormous in these jeans!"

"I have those body freak-out moments sometimes, too. How much does it suck that two such gorgeous, kick-ass ladies are so hard on ourselves?"

Scene 2:

"I don't think I can go to that pool party. There is no sarong big enough and thick enough to cover all the cellulite on my thighs," a pregnant woman complains to her friend.

"Don't worry, you look great. Besides, everyone will be focused on your huge belly!" her friend attempts to reassure her.

Vocab Rehab . . .

"I don't think I can go to that pool party. . . ."

"Come on, your body is doing such *amazing* work. No one deserves a dip in the pool more than you!"

Scene 3:

"I still have so much baby weight to lose! When will all that extra skin on my stomach go away?" a new mother confesses to her friend, also a mom.

"Please, I wish I looked like you!" the friend responds.

Vocab Rehab . . .

"I still have so much baby weight to lose. . . ."

"It's such an overwhelming time, isn't it? How are you dealing with all the changes? How are you feeling?"

It won't be easy and you'll be going against the grain, but you can choose to opt out of the obsession with a target weight gain or weight loss. You can reject the notion that there is a perfect-size bump or a diet or workout plan that you should follow to get your body "back." As a mother-to-be and a new mom, make a new goal for yourself: body confidence. Listen to what your body needs during pregnancy and after. Give yourself time to heal. Confront your fears and insecurities. Redefine your concept of beauty from a place of true health. There is no better time than now.

2

Media Madness: The Truth About Celebrity "Bump Watch" and "Postbaby Weight-Loss Makeovers"

Whether you're an avid tabloid reader or an at-the-salon dabbler, chances are you know a little something about the comings and goings of Hollywood A-listers—especially the ones who are rumored to be pregnant, admittedly pregnant, or just out of the hospital with a new baby. After all, celebrity moms are the new big things. And by big, we mean "Enormous!" and "Still Pregnant!" and "Finally Shedding Her Pregnancy Pounds!" Month by month, we watch these ladies as their bellies and their bra sizes grow. We wait to see what they look like one week after childbirth, then two weeks, three weeks, and beyond. When they are on top of their game, we believe that glamour and Gerber can indeed go hand in hand. When they are caught off guard, we breathe a sigh of relief and give ourselves a break for wearing those ratty old yoga pants for three days straight.

Bump Watch, Preggo Patrol, and Postbaby Weight Loss stories have become much more than superficial star tracking; for the women who follow celebrity news, they provide a universally accepted language for communicating our own fears, challenges, envies, and triumphs.

"The thing we all do with celebrities is comparisons," Janice Min, editor-in-chief of *Us Weekly* told Salon.com. "You really have nothing in common with these people, but in the same way that you want to wear the same shoes and carry the same bag as Kate Hudson, you also think, 'Do I look bigger or smaller than she did at four months?'"

Even when we know logically that stars have more resources than the average woman, we can't stop ourselves from making these comparisons. "Pictures of celebrities just after pregnancy make me jealous. My body changed after the pregnancy, and I know it will never be the same as it used to be. And those famous and sexy women look like they never gave birth," admits Anna, thirty-one.

"It's ridiculous, and yet I can't look away," says Dana, thirty-nine. "It is certainly unrealistic and potentially unhealthy for the average woman to attempt to regain her 'pre-pregnancy shape' within the first six months after the baby. The media rarely goes into the work involved or mentions how these people manage child care while they're working out."

Words and phrases like *ridiculous, unhealthy, frustrating,* and *inane B.S.* came up a lot when we asked women what they thought of the media's coverage of celebrity pregnancy and motherhood. For the most part, it's no secret that celebrities get extra help in the form of trainers, nannies, night nurses, personal chefs, stylists, bodyguards, and other assistants. Unfortunately, our awareness of these extra resources doesn't necessarily reduce the irresistible allure of the baby bump and postbaby weight-loss coverage, or the pressure women feel when they compare themselves to these images. Tempt us with glossy before and after photos and we are like moths to a flame. "I think it's vulgar and completely horrible how no one is off-limits, even during such a personal time as bearing children," says Michelle, twenty-eight. "But I'm guilty of watching the coverage. It's almost like a compulsion—to look at celebrities and see them looking better after a baby than I ever will, even without being pregnant!"

Meredith Nash is an Australian researcher who is exploring how our growing fascination with celebrity pregnancy is affecting nonfamous pregnant women and new moms. She calls her research the Baby Bump Project.

"Every single woman in my study mentioned that getting back into her jeans was a primary goal," says Nash. She has also found that subjects who regularly read tabloids are more likely to describe themselves as "fat" than those who do not follow celebrity culture, and feel heightened pressure to lose their baby weight quickly after delivery. The women we met feel this pressure, too—big time. "It is definitely an issue for me. I see celebrities and how they never look like they gave birth, and I just want to cry," says Lauren, twenty-six.

Images of slim (and often airbrushed) celebrity new moms are giving us a very warped view of what a new mother's body really looks like. "It's gross how the media promote rapid postpartum weight loss, and I know it's ridiculous and unrealistic, but after visiting with relatives who have a four-month-old I realized that those images have affected me; I was surprised to see that the mother 'still' looked kind of pregnant. I was very disappointed in myself," admits Maeve, twenty-five.

The Impossible Celebrity Standard

"If the bump isn't big enough, the celebrities are starving themselves, but if it's too big they're pigging out. And, of course, they're failures if they aren't in a bikini six days after giving birth. If women aren't 'allowed' to have a millimeter of fat on their bodies even in pregnancy and postpregnancy, then it's like we're not allowed to be human."

—Mara, 35

Women Feeling the Pressure

- More than 50 percent of British women admitted feeling pressure to shed their baby weight quickly.
- 90 percent said that celebrity mothers who shed pregnancy pounds soon after giving birth only added to the pressure.

- 16 percent of mothers were so conscious of their body after having a baby that they wouldn't even let their partner see them naked.

- More than a third (36 percent) of new mothers admitted skipping meals in an attempt to lose weight.

Source: 2009 poll of 3,000 British women conducted by Toby Carvery in support of its Healthy Mums program.

The Business of Celebrity Media

Think you can't turn around without reading headlines about how fast the celebrities shed their baby weight? You're right. The number of *People* magazine covers about pregnancy, baby, and postbaby body mentions more than doubled between 2003 and 2005 and has been holding steady ever since. Celebrity magazines are now so desperate to include baby weight stories that they've actually run out of original headlines. In 2008, *US Weekly* recycled "How I Got My Body Back"—once for Trista Sutter in January and then again for Christina Aguilera in June. By August they came up with something new—"How They Get Thin Fast!" (featuring Halle Berry, Nicole Kidman, J. Lo, and Britney Spears). But come October, that one reappeared, this time to describe Angelina Jolie—"How She Got Thin Fast!"

Just as predictable as the reused headlines is the unpredictability of how these magazines praise stars one minute and slam them the next. "It's a strange phenomenon because some celebrities are hailed for accepting their new shapely bodies and others are bashed for not bouncing back sooner," Stephanie, forty, notes. "It doesn't make sense because the tabloids constantly flip-flop between celebrating a pregnant woman's curves and viva-ciousness and condemning postpregnancy weight." It seems there is no way to win this celebrity game. And we would all be wise to remind ourselves that it is just a game.

"For the last two or three years, there's been a massive trend toward pregnancy and baby photos," confirms Stephane Rochon-Vollet, a photographer and fourteen-year veteran in the paparazzi business. With the growth of blogs and online video, the demand for these images is even more intense and immediate. "Between the time that you take the picture to the moment it appears on blogs and Web sites, there can be as little as a thirty-five- to forty-five-minute time lapse," he says.

It's not just the photos that are being sold, either. Like fashion media, tabloids are also in the business of marketing trends to sell products. "I'm in touch with the stores," admits Rochon-Vollet. "You take a picture of any celebrity wearing sunglasses and you can be sure that people all over America will want to buy that same pair. I have a photographer friend who took pictures of Paris Hilton shopping in New York. The following week, a publication printed the name of the store with the photos and they started getting calls. People wanted to know exactly what she bought."

Photographers get paid for taking the photos; stores and brands get paid in eager customers; magazines get paid in advertising, subscriptions, and newsstand sales; blogs and Web sites get paid in traffic that translates into ad revenue; and celebrities, televi-sion networks, and movie studios get paid via the old adage that any publicity is good publicity. All these elements are interconnected and each one relies on the others to survive and thrive.

Celebrity baby and pregnancy fever is now a central part of this profit web. The problem is that what is sold to consumers is the Mommy Brand—the must-have maternity gear and diet and fitness plans—which is a far cry from Mommy Reality.

Read Between the Lines

Any mother will tell you—you can't leave the house without a diaper bag. When you see a charming photo of your favorite celeb with her bundle of joy, see if you can spot the diaper bag on her professionally trained, professionally massaged, and thoroughly moisturized shoulders. If you can't, that means there's another professional carrying that weight around, and she's probably pushing the stroller, too.

We talked to actress Bridget Moynahan, a celebrity mom who is all too familiar with the paparazzi. She told us that what she finds most disturbing about the photos of her that make it into the tabloids is what they *don't* show—the hard work of being a parent.

"I think it's horrible for young girls and women to see all these pictures of celebrities and the way they bounce back or they're strolling around and they have all these nice things," she says. "It's all about how cute the baby looks. It's not that easy and it's not that glamorous. It's not like having the new bag or the new shoe." The focus on the look and the products that go with pregnancy steers us away from the big picture: what it's really like to be a mother.

The confusing messages Moynahan points to are indeed making an impression on young consumers. "I hate all the emphasis put on weight. Like a mother's prime concern postpregnancy should be how well she fits into the thin, conventionally pretty mold. I wish there was more coverage of a mother's thoughts and dreams about her baby, rather than everything always being about looks," says Alya, nineteen.

Thoughts and Dreams, Not Diets and Things

Next time you look at a photo of a celebrity mom and think, *I wish I looked like that* or *I wish I could afford that*, stop and try another kind of dreaming. Look at your child (or your pregnant belly) and think about what kind of future you want to build for him or her. What do you want to accomplish in your life? What kind of mother—what kind of woman—do you want to be?

Secrets of Hollywood Trainers

Celebrities get paid *mucho dinero* to be thin, young-looking, and toned. And they take those fat paychecks and pay other professionals to help them stay that way. For new moms who are part of the Hollywood machine, the pressure is on to get the baby weight off—fast. It is a job requirement for them. And for the rest of us? It becomes an ideal we aspire to.

"Before having kids, I thought, *I'll be like that, too. I'll get back* to running and have my life back," says Audrey, thirty-seven. "But now I realize just how different their lives are from most people's lives. And don't get me wrong: I live a very comfortable, upper-middle-class life with a part-time nanny and a once-a-week housekeeper, plus a babysitter for occasional nights out, and I *still* find it hard—getting up at 6 AM with baby #1, taking care of him, maybe fitting in a power walk with the stroller, breakfast, dressing, working all day three days per week, feeding/bathing baby #1, making dinner, and then eating and going to sleep. And that doesn't include any incidentals like (a) being six months pregnant, (b) having a recurring back problem that's been exacerbated by the second pregnancy and really needs the help of massage/exercise/physical therapy that I just don't have the time for, (c) grocery shopping, socializing or, yeah, um, manicures and pedicures."

Of course, celebrity moms don't just magically get into shape after giving birth; they work out—a lot. They have the professional trainers to guide them through those workouts, full-time child care that allows them to work out practically every day of the week, and personal chefs or food delivery services that ensure they will always have access to nutritious, healthy meals. But before you feel that envy creeping in, let's talk about how much time, energy, and pain really goes into this "getting your body back" business.

Like most women, we did a little "Say, what?" when we heard that Gwyneth Paltrow works out with her trainer, Tracey Anderson, two hours a day, six days a week (in her home gym overlooking the apple orchard and next to the pool so she can hear the kids playing—with the nanny, presumably). Christina Aguilera's workout was detailed in *Us Weekly*; the pop star reportedly worked out ninety minutes a day, five days a week. It would seem that model and actor Milla Jovovich got away with the easiest workout postchildbirth. Her trainer, Harley Pasternak, told *Forbes* that Jovovich got in shape for a movie by working out twenty-five to forty-five minutes a day, five days a week, and by following a designer diet.

To get some of our own scoop, we sat down with celebrity trainer Ramona Braganza in her Los Angeles fitness studio. Braganza trained Jessica Alba and Halle Berry—two of Hollywood's most photographed and talked about new moms—with her program called 3-2-1 Baby Bulge Be Gone. While this program is the basis of the workouts she does with celebrity clients, she admits that there is an "accelerated" version of her plan that she puts into play when there is a deadline (such as a movie/television shoot, a magazine shoot, an ad campaign, etc.) looming. This fast-track plan includes:

1. Twenty to thirty minutes of her program for two weeks, four to five days a week, plus twenty to thirty minutes of cardio on their own.
2. Forty-five minutes of her program for two weeks, five days a week, plus twenty to thirty minutes of cardio on their own.
3. One hour of her program for eight weeks, five days a week, plus twenty to thirty minutes of cardio on their own.

If math isn't your strong suit, we'll spell it out for you. This amounts to at least forty minutes and up to an *hour and a half* of working out five days a week. And when should women start working out after birth? "I leave it up to them. When they're ready, I'm here," says Braganza, who quickly added, "To me, you don't want it to drag out after four weeks. You should get started between two and four weeks if you're not coming out of a C-section." This is not exactly what we were told when we asked an obstetrician the same question.

"With an uncomplicated delivery, a month after the delivery most really active people could resume some level of activity," says Christina Adberg, M.D., an OB/GYN (she advises waiting two to three months after a C-section before doing any exercise besides walking and arm raising). "I never tell people numbers, but if someone has a complicated delivery, they're really not even ready at six weeks. I tell them to just walk. I wouldn't increase their activity level and I'm really careful with the pelvic floor. I wouldn't have them do anything like a squat or a lunge where they could tear their perineum. With a vaginal delivery, it depends on the level of complexity, but no earlier than four weeks have I really seen people resume an exercise routine. And that was only for the fittest people with the easiest deliveries. It can go much longer than that for people who have complicated deliveries."

The difference between the celebrity trainer time frame and the OB/GYN recommendations is just one example of why it doesn't make sense to compare our own lives and our bodies to Hollywood extremes. And besides, if you had the resources to dedicate such an enormous amount of your time to working out so soon after giving birth, would you even want to do it? Looking back, Jessica Alba admitted in an interview for *Elle* magazine that she hated having to get back in shape for a job: "[The workouts] were horrible. I cried. And I haven't worked out since. . . . I'd rather spend an evening with my baby and give her a bath and read her stories and watch her roll around than go work out in a gym." For all her hard work, Alba did look smoking hot in the ad campaign she was trying to get in shape for. But they retouched the heck out of the final photo anyway.

Would You Rather . . . ?

CELEBRITY NEW MOM SCHEDULE	
Monday 6:00–7:30 AM	*Workout*
Tuesday 7:00–8:30 PM	*Workout*
Wednesday 6:00–7:30 AM	*Workout*
Thursday 7:00–8:30 PM	*Workout*
Friday 6:00–7:30 AM	*Workout*

Now what would you do if you could make your own schedule? Choose from the list of options on the next page:

NEW MOM SCHEDULE

Monday 6:00–7:30 AM	*Take a walk*
Tuesday 7:00–8:30 PM	*Daydream*
Wednesday 6:00–7:30 AM	*Take a long shower or bath*
Thursday 7:00–8:30 PM	. . .
Friday 6:00–7:30 AM	. . .

What to do? You can break any of these activities into shorter increments to get the most out of that hour and a half.

- Snuggle with your sweetie
- Sleep
- Read
- Catch up on e-mail
- Call a few friends
- Eat a good meal
- Get a massage
- Daydream
- Pluck your eyebrows
- Upload baby photos
- Workout
- Take a walk
- Write in your journal
- Add cute stuff to your baby's scrapbook
- Take a long shower or bath
- Give yourself /Get a manicure and pedicure
- Tackle your TiVo shows
- Play with your baby
- Shop online
- Research babysitters

Exercise is important for your health. It's something you should incorporate back into your life when your body has healed from childbirth, after you've discussed it with your doctor, and when you feel ready for some activity. If you're itching to get back to intense workouts before you've even had a chance to get a handle on being a new mom, ask yourself where that pressure is coming from. Just because you're hit over the head constantly with the details of every star's postbaby workout plan doesn't mean that those plans are realistic or healthy for you.

"I'm really big on people listening to their bodies in terms of what they can do at a certain time—especially if they've just had a baby," says Teigh McDonough, a new mom, fitness instructor, and founder of SWERVE Studio and Yoga Booty Ballet. "I encourage people to just start strolling around with their baby. It's not the time to get worried about getting your body back. You're dealing with an infant and lack of sleep, so to put pressure on yourself to get back in shape is a mistake. It is way too stressful having an infant in your house to worry about, 'Oh, my God! I don't fit into my size 4 jeans.' I think people drive themselves crazy with that pressure."

In Her Own Words:

The High Costs of Hollywood Pressures

I had this image of women going right back to work and being on set, breastfeeding in their trailers. I put so much pressure on myself to start exercising as soon as I was able to. I was exhausted. I remember I wanted to take a walk up the block and I had a baby nurse at the time and she said, "Lisa, the doctor said it's not enough time." And I almost passed out. I wanted to prove to my manager and my agent that I would be back in shape. I even said that when I first found out I was pregnant. I said, "Don't worry about it. I'm not going to gain a lot of weight. I'll be back in no time."

I was so work-oriented and I had this drive to get in shape, get things back to normal, and start auditioning again. And the funny thing is that I was breastfeeding my child, so I was there, but I just wasn't there in my head. I really regret that now. It's interesting because I thought it was just my profession. But now I talk to my friends who aren't in the business and they're obsessed with their weight and getting back to their prebaby bodies. It's our society.

Lisa Brenner Devlin, actor

Designer Bodies: Mommy Makeovers

It is not our place to knock women who choose to have plastic surgery. That's a personal decision and if you truly believe it's the right decision for you, who are we to judge? With that disclaimer clearly stated, we must say that we find the recent increase in "mommy makeover" plastic surgery procedures nothing short of appalling.

Type the phrase *mommy makeover* into your search engine and you'll find a world of surgeons who promise to provide a "fresh perspective" and a "younger feel." Others are dedicated to the task of helping you "regain the confidence you need to succeed as a mother and as a professional." There is no business training or mommy skill-building involved, though—just a tummy tuck, a breast lift, liposuction, and maybe even some genital "rejuvenation." Because really, what more could our children and prospective employers ask for?

The sales pitch is a familiar one: Look good on the outside and you'll feel better about yourself on the inside. The price tag is steep at an average cost of $12,000–$15,000 for the deluxe combo of procedures that patients pay for out-of-pocket. In our *Extreme Makeover, Dr. 90210* culture, it is easy to find gleeful testimonials from women whose lives have been transformed for the better after going under the knife. We see sad sacks in sweatsuits in the "before" photos and glamorous girls in low-cut gowns in the "afters." What is much harder to find are the stories about how much time it takes to recover from these mommy makeovers, the risks and complications, and the deep insecurities (and histories of disordered eating and serious body image issues) that can lead women to sign up for these surgeries. But when we started digging, we did uncover them.

In a post titled "Fixing Myself?" on theshapeofamother.com, a twenty-two-year-old mother admits that she was diagnosed with anorexia at the age of twelve and suffered with serious postpartum depression after the birth of her daughter. "I absolutely love her and she is my world, but I felt like she 'destroyed' my body. . . . I suffered from severe postpartum depression and ended up being institutionalized for a few weeks. I think the shock of my new body had a lot to do with that. . . . I had a tummy tuck, which I suppose I am glad I did, but had I . . . realized that this sagging extra skin is normal I may not have gone through with it."

Why would any plastic surgeon perform a tummy tuck on a twenty-two-year old mother with a history of anorexia who had been hospitalized for postpartum depression? Good question. And herein lies our biggest issue with the business of plastic surgery. Dollar signs too often trump the glaring warning signs of mental health issues. It's bad enough that obstetricians are rarely aware of their patients' past eating disorders or body image struggles (see chapter 5, Adding Up, Weighing In, and Counting Down), but when women are getting the green light for expensive and dangerous surgeries to "fix" problems that are much deeper than the bumps and bulges they are fixated on, we cry foul. And when these women are mothers—responsible for taking care of their children and teaching them how to value themselves in the world? Well, that's a double foul.

We hope this doesn't sound too cliché, but some of our best friends have been tucked and Botoxed and implanted. Those who haven't done it have hinted that they've thought about it. We still love each and every one of them, even though we haven't made the same choices. We live in a thin-obsessed, youth-obsessed, and perfection-obsessed culture; we understand that it

is not easy for women to resist the calls to "defy" your age and
"reclaim" your body. We have a hard time understanding why
some doctors are offering risky surgical procedures to women who
clearly need to deal with the emotional and psychological issues
that are fueling their body insecurities.

Surge in "Mommy Makeovers"

- In 2006, doctors nationwide performed more than 325,000
  "mommy makeover" procedures on women ages 20 to 39, up 11 percent from 2005, according to the American Society of Plastic
  Surgeons. The increase in "mommy makeovers" over 2005 statistics is more than five times higher than the growth of overall cosmetic plastic surgery procedures (2 percent) during the same period.
- In 2007, The American College of Obstetricians and Gynecologists
  issued a position statement warning against cosmetic surgery of
  the vagina. The group stated that the risks of the procedures out-
  weigh the benefits. Labiaplasty procedures increased 30 percent
  between 2005 and 2006 in the United States. Some women seek
  out vaginal surgery because they are physically uncomfortable, but
  many women do it because they are afraid that their vaginas look
  "old" or they are not "normal"—a fear most often prompted by a
  partner making a negative comment. Instead of questioning the
  partner's reference point (barely legal porn stars), doctors subject
  women to potentially harmful surgery.
- Fifty percent of plastic surgeons say they have patients who have

requested a specific celebrity feature in the last year, including Angelina Jolie's lips and Heidi Klum's nose.

- In 2007, Americans spent $12.4 billon on surgical and nonsurgical cosmetic procedures.
- There was a 137 percent increase in tummy tucks between 2000 and 2007.

Issues and Body Insecurities: The Stars Are Just Like Us

Okay, so they have multimillion dollar mansions and full staffs to help them with working out, cooking, cleaning, shopping, dressing, driving, scheduling, and child care. They take fabulous vacations on the French Riviera, designers send them free clothes, and they get to mingle with other A-listers at catered affairs and extravagant galas. But the truth is that there are plenty of celebrities who stand in front of the mirror and hate what they see. And they've got photographers and critics waiting to confirm that they are indeed "fat" or "ugly" and broadcast it to the world. We know it's hard to muster up much sympathy for people who have so many advantages and perks. For the most part, celebrities choose to be part of the Hollywood machine. They live their lives in the spotlight; scrutiny and criticism come with the package. But a celebrity new mom isn't any less vulnerable or insecure than any other new mom. The fact that everyone is watching her every move (and pound gained or lost) and waiting with bated breath to see when she will "get her body back" actually makes her more likely to feel stressed and inadequate.

Actress Debra Messing appeared on the January 2009 cover of *Shape* magazine to share the details of her weight loss and the shock of seeing herself in the tabloids after the birth of her son in 2004. "On one page it showed all the actresses who got skinny in six weeks or less, and on the other page was me! I was so depressed and frustrated," she told the magazine. She said that it was too difficult for her to manage the responsibilities of being a mother and a working actress with so much working out. She took a slow and steady approach and gradually lost the baby weight.

Of course, the fact that Messing is revealing how hurt she was by the "get your body back" police in an article about how she got her body back is not lost on us. This is how it works in Hollywood. If you want to stay a celebrity, you have to promote your movies and TV shows. You do press junkets, you talk to entertainment reporters, and your publicist works overtime to get you on magazine covers. Baby weight-loss stories sell, so if you're a celebrity mom, you'd better get ready to reveal your diet and workout "secrets."

Celebrity Baby Time Line Tabloid Style

Preannouncement: Photos of celebrity wearing blousey tops. Captions read: "Is it a bump or too many burritos?"

Official Announcement: Pictures of her shopping at exclusive baby boutiques for all the It items.

During Pregnancy: Photos of the growing bump continue, along with comments from tabloid style and beauty "experts" (whom the celebrity has never met, and probably never heard of), explaining exactly which products she uses. Helicopters hover over her baby shower to capture her guests entering and exiting, clutching gift bags filled with [insert product names here].

Delivery Day: When, oh when, will we get to see the baby? Hype and anticipation build to a fever pitch.

Baby Media Debut: Hurray, there is much rejoicing! Mother and baby photo appears on the cover or in the pages of a tabloid magazine. Story makes mention of how mother plans to lose the baby weight. Other publications clamor to make baby weight-loss claims. The *New York Daily News* claimed that Nicole Kidman had lost her baby weight just ten days after she gave birth.

Postbaby Body Advisory Watch Goes into Effect: Please see Hollywood Postbaby Advisory System.

Hollywood Postbaby Advisory System

Day 1–Day 7: Code Green = Low pressure.

Week 2–Month 2 Postchildbirth: Code Yellow = Elevated pressure.

Month 2–Month 3 Postchildbirth: Code Orange = High pressure. We're getting a little anxious if we haven't seen the postbaby diet and fitness "experts" weigh in with their comments.

If there has been no postbaby body red carpet debut or adorable baby photos by three months, automatic *Code Red!*

"I knew as soon as I left the house a week,
even two weeks after giving birth [to daughter Stella],
people were going to take pictures and scrutinize."
—Tori Spelling in *People* magazine

Most of us enjoy an occasional glossy escape to the over-the-top world of glamour and glitter. We laugh at celebrity silliness while simultaneously coveting their ridiculously overpriced ensembles and flawless makeup. We cringe at reality-show train wrecks and wonder what our lives would be like if we were on the A-list. It's all fun and fantasy—until it starts to make us feel bad about ourselves in our real lives. We have to remind ourselves that these images and stories do affect us. Even the smartest and most self-aware women have wished their postbaby bodies were more red carpet–ready, even if there is no red carpet in sight.

"It's a love-hate relationship. I am a smart woman, and I know that beauty ideals in our culture are ridiculously unattainable," says Laura, twenty-nine. "I predict it will be frustrating for me when I'm trying to lose baby weight to see celebs who magically look like they did before pregnancy after an unimaginably short period of time. I have friends who are going through that right now. But on the 'love' side of things, I'm curious about celebrities and their babies, pregnancy wardrobe, all of that."

Sometimes the messages and pressures coming from the media catch us off guard. When we asked Claudia, a fifty-year-old mom, about how she feels about celebrity mothers in the spotlight, she said, "Wow, I barely noticed it—except I guess in the way they wanted me to, which was to think: 'Oh, I didn't get back into shape like that. How could she?' What a sucker I am."

The Phrase: Get Your Body Back

Two things: The key word here is *back*. Let's get something straight. You just had a baby, right? There's no going back. In fact, what you should be thinking about and preparing for is the fact that you are now a parent. The best and, quite frankly, the only option is to move *forward*.

The Phrase: Baby Bump

As in, this whole pregnancy thing is just a bump in the road. Nothing life changing. It also implies that you should be ashamed of your body if your pregnancy is bigger than a bump. "I was incredibly self-conscious about the fact that I didn't have this cute little belly that other pregnant women had," says Amanda, thirty-seven.

The Phrase: Postbaby Body

Uh, where's the baby? This phrase not only conveniently erases that whole childbirth experience, it takes your baby out of the equation, too! Remember, you are a parent now. That party isn't over—it's just getting started. Forget the *post*. You are in the now.

We might all be a lot healthier if we could stop surfing entertainment blogs and buying tabloid or fashion magazines in the
grocery line or at the airport. We might stop comparing ourselves
to those ridiculously unattainable ideals if they weren't in our
faces every day. But there they are. We would have to wear blind-
ers or move to a remote village to avoid the coverage, and we all
know that sometimes those updates about the stars do offer a little
escapist thrill. In the real world, the best we can do is learn to
decode the language of celebrity media and recognize when we're
being manipulated. We can put down the magazines or close our
computers when we feel those twinges of self-doubt, envy, or
annoyance. We can laugh about it, talk about it, write a letter to
the editor, or post our frustrations on a blog. When the stories
about Bump Watch and Celebrity Slim-Downs start to get you
down, remember that there is more to those glossy images than
meets the eye.

Picture Imperfect

Picture the debut celebrity mom and baby tabloid photo. Mother
has the perfect outfit, the perfect hair, and the perfect makeup. She's
blissed out with baby in the perfectly decorated (and spotless!) nursery.
Baby is happily and quietly nestled in mommy's arms, wearing an
adorable (and spotless!) little onesie that perfectly complements
mommy's attire.

What you don't see: The clumps of hair that stayed in the hair-
dresser's brush when he was getting that fantastic mommy's do just

right. The dark undereye circles that the makeup artist skillfully concealed with some superexpensive industrial-strength concealer. The sore nipples that are protected by an antileakage pad in her bra. The Spanx that are probably holding in the jiggle. Maxipads (if the birth was vaginal). Stitches (if the birth was a C-section). The baby puke that was just wiped clean. The poo-filled diaper and the gas that's going to make Junior let loose a major scream in about five seconds.

Baby's inner voice saying: *What the hell am I doing on a photo shoot? Can I get some private time with Mom over here? Call my lawyer!*

3

Let's Talk About Sex (and the) Baby

From **Nine Months** to **Knocked Up,** we've seen endless variations of the same bumbling dad-to-be character. It usually goes something like this: The guy stammers and stutters his way through OB checkups, dutifully sets out on midnight ice cream runs, shrugs haplessly through his honey's hormone-fueled tantrums, gets too freaked out by her pregnant belly to get it on, and then turns several shades of green before fainting in the delivery room.

In real-life relationships, our significant others don't come straight from central casting. Projectile baby vomit isn't always guaranteed comic relief, and failed attempts at pregnancy or post-baby sex are sometimes more frustrating than they are funny. There's no charming indie rock soundtrack that chimes in when you've got hemorrhoids (although, personally, we would love to hear one). The truth is that even when we're able to laugh with our partners about swollen feet and jumbo-size granny panties, we're still thinking "Not sexy!" in the back of our minds—and we're probably wondering if they're thinking exactly the same thing. While it's impossible to know for sure, we can share our own advice and the advice we gleaned from talking to hundreds of women and some of their very candid husbands and partners.

Most couples do have to navigate some "bumps" (so to speak) in the bedroom. Most couples do worry about what will happen to their sex lives and their connection to each other when baby arrives and their bodies and schedules are completely trans-formed. But the changes you'll go through and the emotional highs and lows you'll face together *don't* have to spell curtains for your romance. There are some very important things you need to know about how to hold onto your mama mojo, and we can assure you that none of them involves wearing maternity lingerie or signing up for some brutal exercise boot camp. Every woman is different, and there is no "normal" way to experience your sexu-ality during pregnancy and as a new mother. This is a time when you and your partner will have to commit to staying connected and work together to maintain intimacy in whatever ways feel right for you.

Will I Still Be Sexy When I'm Pregnant?

"My husband doesn't understand my fear of becoming overweight because of pregnancy, but I bring it up sometimes to see what he has to say about it."
—Shannon, 25

"I remind my future husband that I am not always going to have the body that I have today to make sure he is okay with that."

—Jennifer, 27

"I think often about how beautiful I'll look when I'm pregnant, but even though I've come to a much better place about my body, I still worry about what I'll look like after giving birth. My fiancé tries to reassure me that he'll always find me beautiful, but despite my faith in him and my respect for myself, I'm still apprehensive and skeptical."

—Sabrina, 22

"My boyfriend says he will still love me when my boobs are down to my knees because when I laugh it will still be the same laugh that comes out!"

—Jessica, 21

Healthy Body Image Is a Turn-On

You've probably heard that women are harder on themselves than men are on them when it comes to weight and appearance. Lo and behold, that rule also applies for pregnancy and postchildbirth. When we asked dads and dads-to-be to tell us if they had concerns about their partners' bodies, their big concerns were not weight gain or stretch marks (which were at the top of almost every woman's list). Instead, most guys told us they just wanted their partners to feel good about their bodies.

Men Say:

"I didn't have any concerns other than how she would see and feel about her body. She is hard on herself, particularly with regard to weight."

—Kevin, 37

"[My concern was] that she would feel sexy about her body again, whatever the curves happened to be at the moment."

—Josh, 38

"She looks great and gets alarmed about weight gain without real cause."

—Robert, 39

Awww. Lest you think we did our interviews at a Coldplay concert, we should explain that while these guys do sound mighty sweet and sensitive, they've also figured out that this attitude tends to work in their favor. The better their wives and girlfriends feel about their bodies, the better *their* chances of getting some quality (i.e., mutually satisfying) action. Sex is a lot more enjoyable and pleasurable when we're comfortable in our own skin. In other words, bad body image kills the mood. It's like when we're about to get it on, and we reach over to turn off the light because we're embarrassed about how we look.

Joan, thirty-three, admits that her mind has wandered during some very intimate moments with her husband. The bigger her pregnant belly got, the more limited they were in the sexual positions that were comfortable. "I have more issues with my body than I thought I had," she says. "The way we have to have sex now, with me on top, I think, 'Shit, my boobs are sagging.'"

Of course, women's "enormous," "fat," or "sagging" bodies aren't usually the real cause of our problems; it's the fact that we see ourselves through such an unforgiving lens. "I've struggled with body image and eating issues since I was twelve," thirty-two-year-old Jane revealed in her eighth month of pregnancy with her third child. "Honestly, I feel like a blimp. I feel extremely unsexy and have not been able to enjoy being intimate with my husband. . . . I've had zero libido because I feel too self-conscious about how big I am."

Women who have a more positive image of their bodies tell a much different story. "I felt absolutely beautiful and special, because I was! Oh, and the rockin' sex was a bonus," said thirty-two-year-old Sarah, when reflecting on her favorite things about pregnancy. All around the world, pregnant women and mothers are having great sex. These women are not members of some secret society of flawless über babes. They have lumps, wrinkles, and probably some stretch marks, too. They also grasp the simple fact that confidence is the most potent aphrodisiac—and it comes in all shapes and sizes. "Our intimacy is unchanged, and in some ways, it has increased, though the actual act of intercourse has proved challenging as I get bigger and less flexible," thirty-seven-year-old Tanya shared during week 28 of her pregnancy. "We just laugh over this and enjoy ourselves anyway. My husband still finds me very sexy and that makes me feel good."

We do live in the real world and we realize that there aren't many women who go through pregnancy and childbirth feeling completely gorgeous and confident every step (or waddle) of the way. As your body takes on an entirely new shape, all those changes do take some getting used to. You will also encounter physical discomfort, flat-out pain, and plenty of other obstacles that can affect your relationship. But if it's your body insecurities that are consistently preventing you from enjoying sex with your partner, don't assume that things would be smooth sailing if you had a flatter tummy and firmer boobs. You know what they say about the brain being our largest sexual organ? Truer words were never spoken.

Honey, Do I Look Fat?

Hopefully, by this point you have figured out that we are all in favor of open and honest communication. We would, however, like to clarify that we're not so keen on conversations that are doomed to go nowhere. Sort of like this one:

"Does my butt look big in these jeans?" girlfriend asks boyfriend as she's getting ready for their date.

"What? No, you look beautiful. Are you almost ready? We're going to hit traffic," boyfriend responds.

"Really? Because I feel like these jeans are tighter. Don't they look tighter?" girlfriend insists.

Or this one:

"Oh, my God. Why didn't you tell me my upper arms look so flabby?" wife shouts at husband through the bathroom door.

"What? You're crazy. You look beautiful. Are you almost ready? We're going to hit traffic," husband responds.

"No, I have to change. I can't be seen in public wearing short sleeves," wife insists.

Okay, now picture this one:

"Do I look fat?" five months pregnant woman asks her adoring partner.

"Uhhhh. . . . We're going to hit traffic," her adoring partner responds.

Do you see what we're getting at here? Women are in the habit of asking for reassurance from our nearest and dearest. But when they offer that reassurance, we typically ignore them and assume that they are just being nice. Or that they need their vision checked. We don't feel any better about ourselves; they feel cornered. When this pattern continues into pregnancy and motherhood, it's even more of a lose-lose scenario. There's no denying that your body looks different, so the "Do I look . . . ?" questions are just asking for trouble. Plus, don't forget that there is now an extra little pair of ears to absorb all that static. Even if your partner is completely devoted to the task of convincing you that your pregnant body is beautiful, proclaiming sweet adorations from morning until night, those words will fall on deaf ears if you don't believe your pregnant body could be, and in fact is, beautiful. And if you're obsessing over losing those last ten pounds of baby weight, you will likely miss the point when he tells you that he's floored by the incredible feat your body has just accomplished. "Every time I have a little breakdown about my weight, my husband points at the baby and says, 'This came out of you. Look at that! She had to fit in, you clearly had to make room!'" says Sara, a thirty-three-year-old new mother.

New mother Anna, thirty-five, says she is fortunate to have such a supportive partner, but she gets right to the heart of what many other women expressed: "He loves everything that's happening. He loves the shape of my new stomach and breasts. But he'll love anything right now. What's going to happen later? Right now he thinks my maternal self is incredibly attractive, but that doesn't really matter to me because I want to know what everyone else thinks. Does everybody else find me attractive? I hate to admit to such grotesque vanity, but it's there. It's lurking. It's hard to discount it."

This desire to be desired—not just by our partners, but in some larger, universal sense—isn't wrong or shameful. Most of us feel it. Come on, we all know the husbands don't really appreciate the effort we put into that matte red lip we wear on date night. That doesn't stop us from spending twenty minutes perfecting it, does it? We want our beauty to extend beyond what our partners see. We want to know that the rest of the world finds us attractive, too. Motherhood won't automatically erase that craving for outside validation, but it should be the time when we stop hounding ourselves and our partners with the surface questions ("Do I look fat/ugly/old?") that we would never want to hear our children repeat.

"I think I was surprised the most at how supportive my husband is," says twenty-nine-year-old Mackenzie, a new mother. "At first I didn't want him to see my body in my postbaby glory. I worried that it would turn him off, but he doesn't seem to care about anything (or if he does, he's smart enough not to say anything). He still tells me every day how beautiful I am! I think in his eyes, and probably most husbands' eyes, their wives' beauty transforms from something physical, to something more emotional. They think their wives are beautiful for bringing their children into the world—no lumps or bumps or stretch marks could ever change that!"

When your partner sees you through the eyes of love, do not take for granted what a precious compliment you've been given. It's not something to be dismissed or discounted. Do whatever you need to do to see yourself through loving eyes, too (see chapters 4 and 8). After all, we can't teach our children to appreciate their beauty if we don't know how to appreciate our own.

What If He's Just Not That into It?

Before you start thinking we're a couple of Pollyannas, we do acknowledge that not everyone finds dreamy and supportive partners. In fact, some partners don't find pregnancy sexy at all. So who are they and, more important, what are they thinking?

Well, we did encounter a few guys we would immediately put in the Classic Asshole category. These are men who are just generally shaming and critical of women's bodies, whether they're pregnant or not. For these guys, their superficial obsession with women's weight and appearance is really about their own baggage. Their time would be better spent dealing with those issues instead of picking on their partners (see chapter 7, "The WTF Files: How to Deal with Dumb Comments and Stupid Moves").

But we also heard from some otherwise supportive men whose reactions to their partners' bodies could be summed up in two words: *Deer. Headlights.* Remember that you aren't the only one who's probably shocked by how much your body is changing. Most partners can be simultaneously shocked and turned on. But for some it might take a minute, and in a few cases, the shell shock can last longer. This is an especially unfortunate occurrence when pregnancy hormones have you climbing the walls. "My favorite thing about pregnancy was that I was sexually ravenous. My least favorite thing was that my husband was not interested in me," said Willow, thirty-nine. "There are men out there who will still find you incredibly sexy, even while pregnant and after childbirth, even if you gain fifty pounds. Unfortunately, your husband may not be one of them."

Women are accustomed to giving the signs and signals that we're ready for action, and unless he's been running a fever, had a root canal, or was recently kicked in the groin, those signs are usually all it takes to get the party started. It's brutal to be rejected sexually when, according to all popular mythology, you are supposed to be an irresistibly sexy goddess of fertility.

Don't let a few failed attempts at intimacy turn into a gaping distance between the two of you. Confront your partner in as reasonable a manner as can be expected from someone with surging hormones (i.e., avoid hurling any heavy objects). Are there other relationship issues that are causing tension in the bedroom? Resist the urge to take all the blame on yourself ("I must be hideous and unlovable!") or to retreat into silence. Ignoring the problem will only end up making you feel more resentful, which is the last thing you need when you're about to have a baby. Take comfort in the knowledge that you're certainly not the only woman who has found herself in this situation. You will get through it, sexy mama.

The Mechanics: Getting Busy While You're Getting Bigger

Sex during pregnancy is usually perfectly safe, but be sure to talk to your doctor about whether there are any risks or restrictions in your case. If you are told "no sex" get specifics. Is intercourse the only restriction? Are orgasms okay? Is there a time during the pregnancy when sex will be safe again? Once you have the doctor's go-ahead, what happens next? We are going to take a leap here and assume that you don't need a lesson in the basic mechanics. But as your body changes, be prepared for the rules of engagement to change, too. Your tried-and-true boudoir repertoire might need to be adjusted for a variety of reasons, ranging from the physical to the emotional to the hormonal.

Holy Hormones!

Female sexual desire is unpredictable enough in our regular old nonpregnant lives. You ain't seen nothing yet. Pregnancy hormones are a force to be reckoned with. Those smooth moves that were once guaranteed to get you hot and bothered could have you swatting your sweetie away as if you were defending yourself against a sweaty teenager trying to give you a hickey.

"All of a sudden, parts of my body that had been sensitive before were *really* sensitive and you don't touch that!" said Erica, thirty-eight, who told us that sex with her partner didn't come to a grinding halt during her pregnancy, but it definitely slowed down. "Navigating sex in relationships is loaded anyway, and when your body is changing it's like your ground rules are changing." Rachael, thirty-five, said that at week 20 of her pregnancy, she and her husband were still having sex with the same frequency as they were before, but it was different: "My body is very sensitive and uncomfortable now, so my husband has to really take it easy on me."

Hold onto your hats, though. While you might recoil in horror at the idea of being touched sexually one day, the next day (or hour) you could find yourself pouncing on your partner like a porn star. "During pregnancy, your hormones play these tricks on you. You're incredibly horny or you don't want to have sex at all," says Anna, thirty-five. "Sometimes you can say, 'Okay I've been having these crazy orgy dreams for a week now and I've never had dreams like that before.'" Many women reported that their sexual fantasies were more vivid than ever during pregnancy and they found themselves wanting sex all the time. When asked to describe her sex life during pregnancy, twenty-nine-year-old Maren responded enthusiastically, "It was waaaaaay better!"

Pregnancy hormones can also create urges that come on strong and must be dealt with immediately. "I'd be sitting there reading a book and I'd see anything, just the word *sex*, and I'd think, 'Oh, yes. Well, better get on with that!'" remembers

Hermione, forty-four. "I didn't actually want any of the foreplay. In fact, my mantra was, 'Don't touch the rest of my body, and don't touch my boobs. Get to the spot, fiddle with it for two minutes, and be on your way.' I think that was very confusing for my husband. It's more like an itch and you need to scratch it."

He Says:

"The female body suddenly becomes a complete mystery. You think you knew what you were doing, and their nerves just get completely rewired. Suddenly you don't know what you're doing, which is a very awkward feeling. Nothing does what it used to do. You don't trust your touch anymore. You're getting four 'ows' for every 'oh.'"

—Bill, 42, father of two children, with partner for nine years

Is Pregnancy Making You Horny, Baby?

With all those hormones and the increased blood flow down there, some women just can't get enough. Have fun with it. Break out the Hitachi Magic Wand or go have a look at babeland.com!

The Ow Factor

It's not always pregnancy hormones or bad body image that have the biggest impact on your sex life. When you're puking your guts out or struggling to contain the contents of your stomach, nookie is probably the furthest thing from your mind. Back pain, bloating, swelling, fatigue, sciatica, breast tenderness, the constant urge to pee, atomic farts, constipation, hemorrhoids, and the frustrating mechanics of finding workable sexual positions are some of the other wondrous ailments that can cramp your style throughout those forty weeks. "The nausea and sickness kept us from sex for nearly five months, and now I'm so big it's just not very appealing to either of us," Laura, thirty-seven, told us in her twenty-ninth week of pregnancy. We know we're not painting the prettiest picture here, but keep hope alive, ladies. Talk to your doctor about what you are experiencing to make sure you are not suffering needlessly. Ask about your best options for pain relief. Are there any lifestyle or diet changes that might alleviate your specific symptoms? And remember: pregnancy is not a permanent state of being. Yes, the aches and pains you experience will be replaced with new ones as you heal from childbirth—but those won't last forever, either.

Many husbands and partners we talked to said the thing they hated most about pregnancy and childbirth was seeing the person they love suffer and not being able to do anything about it. If there is anything your partner can do to help you, put in your request. Whether it's a meal, a cuddle, or a massage, those gestures build intimacy and break tension, even in the moments when we feel our worst.

Intimacy and Alternatives: Pregnancy Edition

"We have a lot more oral sex."   —Elizabeth, 37

"There were several times where I didn't know how I felt. I didn't know if I wanted to cry, scream, or throw something. It's that little knot where you don't know which spring to pull. So he would make me hot chocolate and something to eat and we would go for a walk. It wasn't focused on how I felt, it was more, 'Let's go do something together to distract you.'"   —Mary, 31

"I think we communicated well and we also were very intimate with each other—taking showers together every day, touching each other, being close. This is not to say we weren't having sex—we just weren't having a lot of sex."   —Erica, 38

"He would do little things, like one day he went to a salon and talked this woman into coming home with him to give me a pedicure because I was on bed rest with twins and couldn't leave the house. He did things like that because he knew I was feeling really gross at home and I couldn't do my feet myself because I couldn't reach them."   —Kristen, 34

"He wants to have sex with me, but if I am not into it (which never happens!), he is okay just to snuggle. He likes to rub my belly and sing to my belly. He always wants to touch me, even in small ways— having my feet on his lap on the couch, having our legs touch in bed, always insisting on time to spoon in the morning before we get up."   —Erica, 32

"When I'm not thinking about [my husband], I think about movie stars. I just create my dreams."   —Joan, 33

We're Not Alone

Some expectant couples get spooked when they think about the fact that it's no longer just the two of them in the bedroom. "I think my husband sometimes feels like he is going to hurt me or the baby might know what is going on," said Elizabeth, thirty-seven, whose fear was expressed by both dads and moms-to-be. Jessie, thirty-four, told us that she had to get past the idea that there was an extra little person who could now be privy to the goings-on. "It was weird for a while because I felt strange having sex with a baby in there, but I'm over that and things are good again." Experts agree that your baby won't be able to see anything or have any clue what you're up to. Carry on!

The Main Event: A Spectator Sport?

Are husbands traumatized by watching birth? Will your partner have to go through special vagina reintroduction training to have sex with you again? Well, there was that one guy who appeared on an episode of *Oprah*, which no less than ten people e-mailed us about (yes, we saw it!). Of course, we don't doubt that this case was very real and very difficult, and there may well be a whole cadre of vagina-phobic husbands out there. We must tell you that we haven't met any of them. What we did learn is that women and men usually have opinions about the "to watch or not to watch" question *before* they ever set foot in the delivery room. If they discuss their fears, expectations, and levels of squeamishness together, that's usually the best way to head problems off at the pass. Of course, no plan is set in stone when it comes to birth, but it is a good idea to communicate what you're okay with and listen to what your partner is okay with. "I've been with dads who didn't want to see it and they just stayed up by the mother's head," says Sherry Rumsey, a doula and student midwife who practices in Los Angeles. "Some want to see, and they want to touch the baby's head as it's crowning and they want to be there completely. For other dads, that's just a little too much birth for them. You have to respect where they are and what level they want to be involved."

To Watch or Not to Watch

The great thing about men is that no matter what side of the fence they're on, they seem to have a true knack for delicate phrasing and, ahem, flowery language.

"It's not my place. I shouldn't be there," says Fred, a 47-year-old husband and father of three who was absolutely certain that he did not want to watch his wife give birth. "My friends who watched their wives deliver tell me, 'Oh, it's incredible.' I'll say, 'What kind of incredible is it? Can you specify that?' Then they're stuck and I'll ask them to explain the whole pushing thing. 'Is that beautiful? Because if you want, you can watch me take a big shit!' And then they'll admit, 'Yeah, you're right. It's terrible, but we can't say that.' Of course we can't say that! But for real, I don't want to be in there."

Eugene, 42, watched his daughter being born by C-section. He said he gained a new appreciation for his wife's strength, and, like a true guy's guy he found a way to compare the experience to a blockbuster action movie: "It was like watching **Alien!** You're so proud of your wife. I told her it was fucking amazing."

There are plenty of partners who sign up for a front-row seat and their enthusiasm for the lady bits does not wane, regardless of what they see. "My labia were swollen, I was twice my normal body weight with the water retention, and I had an enormous episiotomy cut. I was basically splayed open like a side of beef. Then my husband really wanted to have sex with me two months later," recalls Tina, forty, who delivered twins. "I had an epidural and I remember him looking between my legs during the birth and looking at me and saying, 'You didn't feel that?' He got over it really fast. Maybe I just have a really forgiving husband. If a man feels that's going to affect him, he's usually not going to look. I'm of the belief that men are just so happy to get some that they don't care what it's ever looked like."

Sarah, thirty-two, says her husband doesn't like blood and was nervous about the birth. "[He] thought that maybe he would just stay up at my head. But I think it was just such an amazing sight to see a little human appear that he couldn't help but watch. There was a good deal of blood and he said that this left an image in his mind that was kind of scary. He watched me get a few stitches, too, so that didn't help." Her husband was not turned off forever, though. Once he was sure she was healed, he was good to go. "He just kept checking in with me and when I felt pretty good, then we started having sex again."

Some women are sure they don't want their partners to watch, and some are sure they do. Partners might have equally strong feelings one way or the other. And then there is the middle ground, where feelings aren't so clear-cut. "I'm still kind of split about the whole situation because I was very grateful that he was there," says Anna, thirty-five. "He was incredibly helpful and I think it was good for him to have seen his daughter being born. It was great because he held her right away. I still had to have work done and I wanted her to be held and not taken away. But for me—I didn't want to be seen like that. It was completely humiliating! No, not attractive. Not sexy. Yes, we're partners. We're parents together. But I prefer to have my humiliating moments on my own. I don't need witnesses."

Birth is messy and primal (obvious statement of the century)—modesty usually goes out the window when you're in the midst of it. Your partner could end up seeing more of you than you ever imagined you were capable of revealing. As long as that exposure isn't happening against anyone's will, have faith that your sex life will return again.

Finding Your Way Back into the Groove

Let's be honest. Bringing a newborn home will be a handful. You're probably not going to be breaking out the negligee and doing a striptease by candlelight anytime soon. As a couple, your first task will be to get a handle on the madness. "I think dads and moms can have a very Disney idea of what it's going to be like after the baby comes and the reality can be a big shock. A newborn is demanding and takes so much time to feed, bathe, change, burp, and get to sleep. It can be a very exhausting process to get through those first weeks. Postpartum can be a big shock for both partners," says Sherry Rumsey, a doula and birthing class instructor.

Take the time *you* need to rest and to heal. You'll need to get the official okay to go back to having sex after delivery, which usually happens at your six-week checkup. Most doctors say six weeks is enough healing time for vaginal deliveries and C-sections with no complications. Some women we talked to were excited and curious to try it as soon as they got the thumbs-up; others told us they were afraid of the pain or they just weren't ready. If your partner has that six-week date circled on the calendar, you would be wise to offer a friendly reminder that many women need more time—and you might be one of those women. Without the heads-up, it could become a looming issue in the relationship, should the date pass with no intercourse. We say *intercourse* here because there are plenty of other ways to be intimate. In fact, creativity, connection, and a broader definition of sex will go a long way when you're trying to reconcile your life as a couple with your new life as parents.

So It's Been Six Weeks . . .

"I might have said something about how there was no way, no how until the stitches were well and truly healed!"   —Merri, 25

"[Sex] felt so great (OK, physically not for the first few times back)
but emotionally and eventually physically it was great to connect and
have 'me' time by having 'us' time that you can get nowhere else."

—Jen, 38

"This whole thing about wait six weeks is absolutely rubbish. We
tried it at eight weeks and it was so painful we couldn't carry on. We
finally managed later at twelve weeks. For me it was still quite
painful and I had a regular vaginal birth. If you're told six weeks,
and that's what you expect, you may be a bit disappointed when your
body just did this amazing thing."   —Sarah, 32

"After five weeks I was very keen."   —Nicole, 32

"I was eager to try it, but it was really weird. I had to use tons of lube
until I stopped pumping [breast milk] and then I was back to my
normal self. At six weeks, they said it was okay, but ow! I think I was
also really wide. I kept asking, 'Are we doing it? Ow! Are we doing
it? Ahh!' I think we were both really nervous that it would be like
that from then on. But every time after that was better. Maybe that's
where they want you to start so you'll be really happy the next time!"

—Amy, 37

Magali says:

"I was very, very curious about making sure that all was still in proper
functioning mode down there. That said, I was absolutely petrified at the
idea of pain. Birthing my daughter was a whole new level of intense

pain, and after six weeks I hadn't forgotten any of it. The fear of feeling any beginning of discomfort made the experience more of a nervous fiddle than a relaxed reuniting. I felt like a virgin again, trying to find what worked and what didn't feel good. I felt completely inexperienced and insecure about my own body."

Hey, What About Me?

Now that a little person suddenly needs you for *everything*, it also means that a certain someone else is not getting the same amount of attention. Guess who? The partners we talked to said they did miss sex in those months after the baby was born, but that wasn't what bothered them the most. The issue that seems to cause the biggest relationship rifts is a little something we like to call New Mother Tunnel Vision. "I didn't understand until later that it is much greater than sex. It's jealousy, not over the woman's body, but over how the baby is consuming all of the woman's body and attention. If you are breastfeeding, you can spend hours upon hours each day doing nothing else. There is quite literally no physical access to the woman. But it is more than that. The baby is taking up all my physical attention and that makes him feel excluded. That's what happened in my relationship," explained Sarah, thirty-two. When your every waking hour is consumed with caring for your newborn, other people can easily fall out of focus.

He says:

"Guys have way more patience than women think. We can wait [for sex], but you need to show something. . . . The 100 percent love she had for me can't turn into 90 for the baby and 10 for me—it has to be 100 for me and 100 for him! And for her, at the time, I'm telling you, it was 99 for the baby and I was 1 percent. In the morning I would have the baby in my arms, she would come down the stairs and see the baby, take the baby from me, say hi to the baby. And to me? Nothing! My guy friends all say it's the same for them. I talked to my wife about it. Now we have a rule. I get a good-night kiss every night, even if she's too tired for anything else. I'm at least getting that." –Fred, 47

Tension can also arise when new mothers start to believe that no one else on the planet could possibly be trusted to take care of their babies—including their partners. "There is a certain anxiety that sinks into your stomach. You feel like an animal, you want to protect that baby, and you think that you are the only one who can do it right," remembers Peggy, thirty-two. "You have to fight that, because otherwise you get a little loopy and there is a sort of competition that develops with your husband."

Dina, thirty-four, had a similar experience. "My mother-in-law and my mother both told me that I just have to leave [my husband] with the baby and a bottle and just go. I did that for the first time recently and it was *really* hard. I thought it was hard for him, and that was my perception at the moment—that he can't deal and he doesn't want me to leave. We got in a fight the next day and he said to me, 'You don't trust me.' And I thought he didn't want me to leave him with the baby. He was like, 'You couldn't even leave!' And I realized that it was my issue, too. I was really nervous about leaving."

Take the Time and Take Your Time

Caring for baby can result in otherworldly exhaustion. Your hours are devoured by feedings, diaper changes, and piles of laundry that never seem to diminish. Your world shrinks to the square footage of your bedroom, kitchen, and bathroom, and yet somehow you feel as if you're running some kind of Iron Mom triathlon every day. Fatigue like this moves sex pretty far down your list. "Where is the time? We both are exhausted. It has come up but we end up falling asleep first," says thirty-one-year-old Mary.

Are you tied to the romantic notion that you must have spontaneity to have a passionate relationship? Get over that now. Welcome to the world of parenthood, where if you don't pencil in quality time with your partner, it might not happen at all.

Hermione, forty-four, planned a brief afternoon outing for her husband's birthday three weeks after giving birth to their first son. They took a drive in the mountains and pulled off the side of the road for a nice, scenic . . . blow job. Hey, remember what we said about creativity? We weren't kidding. But Hermione says the scheduling that made the biggest impact on her marriage post-baby had nothing to do with physical intimacy. She made a standing weekly lunch date with her husband after her first son was born. "Every single Wednesday, I would get dressed up. He would be on the other side of town, meet me halfway, and we'd go to a nice restaurant. I'd take the baby so he would get to see the baby during the day and he would get to see me. We would only meet for an hour, but we connected. For a small thing to do, it was really effective."

It's true that you won't have a lot of energy to give as a new mom, but keep in mind that even the most minimal amount of time and effort can go a long way in keeping your relationship healthy.

Intimacy and Alternatives: New Mom Edition

"In the beginning, the whole thing was overwhelming and sex was not even in the stratosphere. We were sleeping with clothes on, which we don't often do, because we had to get up every hour and a half to try to feed the kid. Finally, after a couple weeks of that, [my partner] was the one who said we need to start sleeping naked again and bring that back into our relationship." —Erica, 38

"I think that two months after giving birth, you should go away for two days with your husband. Every time [my husband] and I left for a weekend in a hotel, we were making love like rabbits. It got expensive but it worked!" —Peggy, 32

Since a weekend away isn't always financially feasible or realistic, it's important to make the most of your friends and family network of babysitters. Even just a few hours of quality couple time (even if it's not in bed) helps!

Back Away from the Boobs!

Women who breastfeed often lose interest in sex, and that can happen for several reasons. First, there is a very practical medical explanation. Prolactin, the milk-producing hormone, inhibits the release of estrogen (the hormone that gives us a libido). "[They] may notice that their girl parts don't look the same as they did in the past," says Barbara Dehn, a women's health nurse-practitioner. "The labia shrink and things are a little dry. This isn't from a vaginal birth, because it happens for women who had a C-section, too. What happens is that Mother Nature doesn't want women to be hot for their partners too soon after giving birth. For that baby to have enough milk to survive, it's essential that the mom not enjoy sex and make another baby, which would decrease milk supply." Damn, Mother Nature. Give a girl a break. Though the human race has evolved to circumvent this biological occurrence with handy inventions like K-Y, getting juiced up on the outside doesn't always mean you'll be in the mood.

Some breastfeeding mothers also described the feeling of being "touched out." When you've got a little one sucking on your nipples all day long, you might not be too excited when your partner wants to take a turn. "You have these juicy big tits and they really want to go for them, they just want to play with them," says Hermione. "So you're dangling these toys in front of their face, but anybody who goes toward your nipple you basically want to punch. It was hard because I used to try to redirect my husband and say you can massage them, play with them, but if you touch the nipple, I will kill you! And it was very confusing for him because he was very nervous. It becomes like a minefield."

He says:

"If I came within five feet of her breasts, the National Guard would be ordered. Which was kind of a nightmare. [It] makes you very sexually confused."

—Bill, 42

Elita is a thirty-year-old breastfeeding mom who created the blog Blacktating (Blacktating.blogspot.com). She says that breastfeeding did knock her libido out for a while, but she wants new moms to hang in there and give themselves time to get back to feeling sexy. Her breasts are part of her sex life again, and they also continue to nourish her thirteen-month-old son: "We need to embrace both functions of our breasts. I can't be bothered to be embarrassed if my milk comes down and I leak during sex or orgasm. My man has seen me give birth so I am not sure what could shock him at this point. Are leaky breasts that big of a deal? When my son is nursing I am not thinking about sex and when I am having sex with my partner, I am not thinking about breast-feeding my son."

Remember Your Oxygen Mask

When you plan to have a child with your partner, remember that you also need to plan for how your life will be transformed as a couple. In a February 4, 2009 *New York Times* op-ed titled "Till Children Do Us Part," author Stephanie Coontz makes the point that couples who go into parenthood with a plan for how they will keep their relationship strong postbaby fare much better than couples who fall into parenting with no plan. She cites psychologist Jonathan Coleman: "The airline warning to put on your own oxygen mask before you place one on your child also holds true for marriage." Intimacy with our partners—both physical and emotional—is truly the breath of our relationships.

Jen, thirty-eight, says her sex life isn't perfect or effortless, but she recognizes how it keeps her connected to her husband. "Sometimes it is awkward and difficult and doesn't always feel fantastic . . . but it keeps you laughing, playing, and surmounting challenges as a couple in a way you don't do with anyone else. For us, it is the secret of survival during these nutty raising-young-kids years."

Pregnancy and motherhood will reorder your life in every way imaginable. The changes to your body, your image of yourself, and your sexual desire will impact your relationship—and that impact will probably be different, depending on the minute, month, or year. Talk about these changes, do your best to plan for them, and navigate them together with a sense of humor and a deep respect for each other.

4

New Addition, New You: Style & Beauty for Expectant and New Moms

Women have clear ideas about how we define beauty and style for ourselves. Whether you spend two minutes or two hours on your makeup application, $20 or $200 on a pair of shoes, you know what time and money you're willing to invest in your beauty routine and what you can't be bothered to deal with. There is a sense of pride in the style and beauty choices you make and no matter how superficial, they are part of your identity. Perhaps that is why there is so much anxiety about what will happen to those choices when a baby enters the picture.

Will you be basking in the angelic glow of pregnancy in gauzy, goddess gowns, or will you turn into a hormone-crazed maniac hobbling around in a muumuu? Will you be the mom in cute strappy sandals or the mom in, gulp, mom jeans? "I'm scared that I'll be stuck as a lumpy, postpregnancy woman after the big priority shift. You know, that moment where it is no longer okay to think or care about yourself," said Caroline, twenty-seven. Relax, we're here to tell you that while your beauty and style regimen will go through some changes, that doesn't mean you'll end up wearing pants with "nine-inch zippers and casual front pleats," as advertised on *Saturday Night Live*.

Beauty Routines

"I wear makeup every day (foundation and everything), do my hair every day (about 20 minutes), I wax, get mani/pedis, and get laser. And for some reason, I don't feel high maintenance."   —Liz, 29

"I'm low maintenance. I wear eyeliner, brow liner, powder, and lip balm. I buy clothing that's stylish, but always it's bought on sale and may not reflect current trends. I love vintage."   —Christina, 29

Beauty & Style During Pregnancy and After Baby . . .

Seventy-five percent of mothers we surveyed told us that their style and beauty regimens had changed since they became moms, and sometimes in ways you might not expect.

"What's a manicure? Oh God, how I miss being pampered!"

—Coni, 36, mother of a 2-year-old

"I enjoy taking care of myself. Spa treatments and mani/pedis make me feel good. When I'm taking care of myself, I can take care of my family. It's frustrating when coworkers say that you don't need to dress up because you are married and have a kid. Translation: no one is looking at me now that I'm a mom. Or that being a mom has now made me unattractive, so why bother even getting up to brush my hair."

—Taiia, 35, mother of a 7-year-old

"I spend far less time and money shopping and doing 'pampering' now. This is partly because I have less disposable income. But I look at it as temporary and that in a few years, I will gradually regain some of that 'freedom' that came with treating myself to things related to vanity. I do still believe in allowing myself small luxuries, and I get massages and pedicures sometimes, or I walk with a friend, or go to the grocery store alone (!) when my kids are in child care. Funny what I consider a luxury now."

—Jenni, 38, mother of a 2-year-old and a 7-year-old

"Before I was a mom, there wasn't a day you'd find me without full makeup on and my hair done. I was fashionable, trendy, trim, and shopped all the time. . . . But as time passed, I realized that in terms of priorities that was closer to Z than A. I am now struggling to find the happy medium between my [beauty] regime and my responsibilities. You don't have to be perfect. I feel loved, lovely, and special with the smile from that baby—makeup or no makeup."

—Sarah, 28, mother of a 3-year-old and a 10-month-old

*"I'd love a haircut and facial, I just haven't had enough pumped milk
to leave the house for long enough."*

—Kate, 35, mother of a 3-month-old

Motherhood is a new phase of your life—one that will absolutely have an impact on the beauty and style decisions you make. But that's not necessarily a bad thing! Hopefully, your look has already been evolving over time. Our looks certainly have. Claire retired her combat boots and polyester butterfly-collar shirts after college (think *That '70s Show*, except it was the '90s). Magali has not been spotted in her African print pants or any of her cowboy *hats* (yes, that is cowboy hats, plural) any time recently. There's no going back to some of the looks we've sported. We wouldn't want to, and neither would anyone who cares about us even one iota. They were part of what made us who we were at the time. Now we prefer to walk around with a style that reflects who we are *today*. The truth is that there's really no such thing as "dressing like a mom"—it's all about dressing like who *you are* as a mom. Your life will be different and your body will different, so think of pregnancy and new motherhood as one of those opportunities for a beauty and style evolution.

Your Pregnancy Style Primer

Even though weight gain and pregnancy go hand in hand, it can still sting when your clothing starts to become a glaring reminder of those extra pounds you're packing on. Some women are so excited about pregnancy that they're skipping to the maternity stores, but we talked to many, many others who were unsettled by the prospect of elastic waistbands and larger sizes. Wherever you fit on the spectrum, there are some basic steps you can follow to express your unique style throughout your pregnancy.

Don't Sweat the Small Stuff

Do you harbor the fantasy that you will be one of those adorable pregnant women who gets away with wearing her low-rise jeans up through her second trimester? We hate to be killjoys, but it's probably not going to happen. One of the kindest things you can do for yourself is to pack up anything that would qualify as "form-fitting" immediately. This is a surefire way to avoid the agony of trying to squeeze into something that's too small. You can keep the oversized cardigans and roomy blouses, but if you have any articles of the skinny jeans or tiny tops variety in your wardrobe, they should go. And we're not kidding about packing it up. Put those clothes in a box, and seal it up tight. Personally, we advise you not to open that box again until at least a year after you've given birth. You know what they say about nine months to gain the weight, nine months to take it off? Well, we're adding a few extra months for good measure. That's a lot of seasons in fashion-speak, so chances are good that you won't even be interested in some of those clothes once you dig that box out again.

Magali says:

"I had these great baggy, boyfriend-style jeans that I thought I could continue to wear as 'maternity jeans.' Well, that was an ill-conceived plan. I kept trying to make them work to the point where every time I was sitting down I was unbuttoning the top button because they were so uncomfortable and I repeatedly would forget to rebutton them when standing up. Needless to say, it was not a good look! And it didn't feel so great, either. So spare yourself and those around you. I've been there and won't go back again."

If you are one of those clothes collectors who could wear a different outfit every day of the year if she wanted to, you will need to get used to the "less is more" idea during pregnancy. Unless you have an unlimited budget, pregnancy and motherhood will force you to rely on a smaller rotation of pieces.

As a rule, the same pair of maternity pants or maternity jeans paired with three different loose-fitting tops will do your figure a lot more favors than three different, too-tight-but-still-trying-to-squeeze-into-'em pants worn with those same three tops. More variety does not mean more flattering. Get the ill-fitting or soon-to-be-ill-fitting stuff out of your way and start focusing on adding simple, comfortable basics you can dress up. Take it from the Frenchies, who know their style. The three secrets to looking chic are (1) a great haircut; (2) a beautiful bag; and (3) some gorgeous shoes. You really don't need to have endless clothing options.

Do Some Preemptive Shopping

Prone to dressing room meltdowns? We urge you to buy a few cheap but stylish basics in bigger sizes before you need them. Conventional wisdom is that you shouldn't invest in too many clothes too soon because you can't predict how much or how fast you will grow. We agree about not investing too much money, but we're going against the grain to say that you *should* have some larger pieces in waiting. And here's why: It's a lot more fun to have new things you're excited to wear hanging in your closet than to be running out to the store in desperation because you can't squeeze into anything you've got. The "I'm too big for everything I own!" mind-set does not make for happy shopping. Imagine being told that you have to try on string bikinis when you've got PMS. Yeah, it's kind of like that. So spare yourself the misery and pick up some inexpensive and versatile items in several sizes up from what you usually wear—especially if you know that going into a dressing room with those bigger and bigger sizes is going to be tough on you. It's okay to get some things that you can grow into in the privacy of your own home.

Spend Wisely

As sick as we are of the incessant Hollywood Preggo Patrol, the one positive thing we heard from women about all the media coverage is that they find it comforting to see so many examples of pregnant style done right. "The only good thing I see about pregnant celebs is the clothes they wear when they're pregnant," says Erica, thirty-three. "Seeing celebrities looking fantastic in outfits that aren't those hideous tents of yesteryear makes me love the idea of dressing up and truly glowing. [They] have made it okay to revel in how you dress your bump." It is true that we've come a long way from the maternity muumuus. Of course, most women don't have a celeb-sized bank account to buy a designer maternity wardrobe. "It's hard to find maternity clothes that are both decent-looking and affordable, so a lot of times I wind up looking frumpy," said thirty-two-year-old Joanna in her thirty-fourth week of pregnancy. Here's how to get the most bang for your buck.

Where to Spend:

- ✓ **A pair of black maternity pants** that you can wear to work and out for an evening. It's worth it to go for quality on this purchase. Black pants are versatile and you'll get a lot of mileage out of them.

- ✓ **At least one pair of good maternity jeans** or track down a hand-me-down pair from a girlfriend or secondhand boutique. If you buy yours new, don't forget to offer them to a friend when you're done with them. You can always ask for them back if you need to bring them back into your rotation!

- ✓ **Dresses.** If you're looking for clothing that will work for office and evening, dresses are your best bet. Treat yourself to one special-occasion dress. "One of the things I bought was a really cute dress. It was a fun dress, like a party dress. I was psyched about it, and that makes a difference," said Erica, thirty-eight. Wrap dresses, A-line cuts, and empire-waist styles give you room to grow, and they'll still look great after you've given birth. If you're rocking the dresses in the winter, pick up some pretty tights (size grande for your grande tummy!) and pair your look with boots for versatility.

- ✓ **Bras.** Remember, it's not just your breasts that are expanding. Your whole torso will get wider. You will go up in bra size at least a few times during your pregnancy, and this is not where you want to skimp. There are enough physical discomforts you'll have to deal with, so why add another one to the mix by not treating your growing girls to the support they deserve? Do your bra shopping at a store where you can get fitted, preferably a place that specializes in maternity bras. Leave this task to the pros. It will be time and money well-spent.

Where to Save:

Accessories. You'll have fewer clothing items to work with, so add some variety with your accessories. Go for it with the shoes, bags, belts, and jewelry, ladies. These are your pregnancy style essentials! The good news is that you can work with what you've already got (there's no such thing as "maternity accessories"), and you can continue to do so after pregnancy. If you do want to pick up some new stuff, it's certainly not hard to find inexpensive costume jewelry. Web sites like etsy.com offer a wide selection of unique, handmade accessories. You can also pick up cheap, chunky necklaces at Forever 21 and other affordable chains. We think they're the perfect complement to a big belly.

Tops. While you can't avoid the maternity stores if you want to find jeans or pants of the nonyoga variety, it is easier to circumvent the maternity markup when you're shopping for tops. Look for longer, roomy shirts that will accommodate your growing belly. Raid your partner's closet for some classic button-downs you can dress up with belts and jewelry.

Comfies. Yoga pants and oversized T-shirts might not be the pinnacle of high fashion, but we would be lying if we didn't tell you that they are an easy, affordable, and um, comfortable option—especially when your body gets more unwieldy in those last few months of pregnancy. Oh, we can almost feel the wrath of Stacey and Clinton as we type this. We hope they'll forgive us. "I want to be comfortable and mobile and flexible, as I am still chasing a toddler around," said Amy, thirty-one, in her eighth month of pregnancy. "I have succumbed to the stretch pants. Not high fashion, but they are soft and they work, and I haven't purchased a single piece of maternity wear."

Like Something in Black? Get It in Blue, Too

This style rule isn't exclusive to pregnancy, but if you haven't already gotten into the habit of applying it, now's the time. When you find a piece that gives you confidence and it just feels like *you*, make your life easier and get it in a few colors. Many women told us they had a go-to, "signature" item they wore during their pregnancies. "I had to get through winter in my second pregnancy and I found that extremely difficult," says Hermione, forty-four. "Most things were too short, and I would get this cold gap on my belly. I found one shirt that was cut so it covered my belly completely. I got it in nine colors and then I could put a cardigan on top."

Pregnancy Style Tips from a Fashion Editor

We asked Marlien Rentmeester, West Coast bureau chief of *Lucky* magazine, to share her style tips for pregnant women. This is a topic she knows well—we interviewed her when she was four months pregnant!

Shop vintage. "It's so inexpensive, it's deeply chic, it's one of a kind, and it's not the sort of thing that you would see on everyone else. You can make a real statement that way. And you can alter it, too."

Think proportions. "Clothing that's too tent like actually makes you look bigger than you are. If you wear something big, maybe belt it, or pair it with a fitted sweater so you have some balance. It gives a shape and streamlines you."

Stay true to your style. "One of the best pregnancy outfits I ever saw was on a woman who was wearing a dress that she had obviously bought when she was not pregnant. Nonetheless, she wanted to wear it, so she wore it! She put a slip under it and then she unbuttoned the buttons at the belly. Somehow, it just worked on her. It might have looked crazy on someone else, but I thought the fact that she wanted to maintain her style made her look stylish."

Looking for Vintage? Check Out:

Ebay.com

Rustyzipper.com

Mamastonevintage.com

Wide Load Underwear

It's not just your bump that grows during pregnancy—so does your rump. "One of my least favorite things about pregnancy was constantly having to buy bigger underwear," says Kate, thirty-five. We hate to break this to you if you're newly pregnant, but it won't be long before those sexy cheekies will barely cover one cheek. So resign yourself to the fact that your panties, like the rest of your wardrobe, will have to be upsized, too. And please do yourself a big favor and get *cotton* panties that allow for maximum air circulation. Pregnant women are prone to yeast infections, so don't push your luck by putting anything synthetic near your lady parts.

Magali's Maternity Essentials

1 black drawstring skirt

2 pairs of yoga pants (one drawstring, one elastic waist)

Indian tunics in every color

1 hand-me-down little black dress

1 pair of hand-me-down maternity jeans

2 dresses I wore later in the pregnancy (one halter-style, one wrap dress)

Cardigans and shawls. My body temperature was changing constantly, so I always dressed in layers I could peel off when I started to feel warm!

2 va-va-voom, hello cleavage! bras at the beginning, 4 sports bras (2 white, 2 black) for the middle, 3 nursing bras (black, white, and beige) for the end of pregnancy, which I wore until I stopped breastfeeding

Don't Let the Sizes Weigh You Down

For sanity's sake, pregnancy is a time when you must let go of your attachment to a specific clothing size. As someone who is about to become a mother, your sense of self-worth cannot hinge on whether you can fit into whatever size you think is "ideal" for you. Is that a belief you would ever want your child to absorb? What's really ideal is to find clothes that are flattering, comfortable, and versatile. Sizes always vary from store to store, so don't have a heart attack if you end up wearing sizes that seem beyond what you ever imagined you would wear. That goes for pregnancy, and it applies for after delivery, too. "I almost didn't purchase anything because the numbers scared me so much. I can't get past that number thing," says Sara, a thirty-three-year-old new mom. "I've always said to myself that my goal was never a weight. My goal was always a size when I was dieting. So now that I'm stuck in sizes that are much bigger, it's really started to make me cringe."

The number on the scale doesn't define any of us, and neither does that number on the tags of our clothes. If it's making you that miserable, take a pair of scissors and cut those labels out of sight and out of mind.

Belly Photos: Behind the Scenes of Pregnancy Photography

Are you ready to be America's Next Top Preggo? A good photographer can capture an image that allows you to have a special visual keepsake of your pregnancy. "When you photograph a pregnant woman, there are so many things she is usually self-conscious about. Women will come in and warn me, 'Oh, there are stretch marks on my stomach, my butt, or my belly,'" says Alvera Taheri, a photographer who specializes in pregnancy photography. But even for women who feel insecure about their appearance, the photos and the experience of having them taken can actually be a confidence booster.

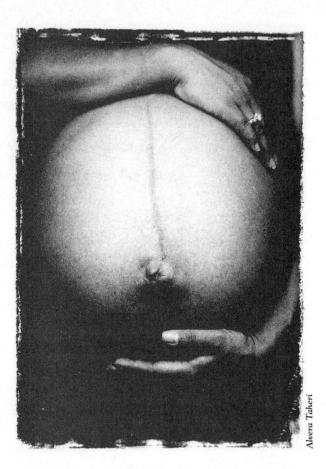

Alvera Taheri

Q: When is the best time to get my photo taken?

Wait until you're visibly pregnant, but don't put it off until you're too close to your delivery date! "I usually like to do it around seven to eight months because by the end women are usually really big and uncomfortable. You would be surprised how many last minutes I get: 'I'm due next week and I really want to take a picture!' I get those so often, I can't even tell you," Taheri says.

Q: Where should I do the photo shoot?

Taheri prefers to do photo shoots in women's homes, where they are most comfortable: "I encourage women to do it in their own homes, in their bedroom, where they made the baby. I'll set up the backdrop there. I've noticed a huge difference with those photos. It makes them so relaxed."

Q: Was that really me?

Looking at your pregnancy photos after you've given birth can bring up a whole host of emotions, but the one Taheri sees most frequently is shock: "Women come in to look at their pictures after they've given birth and they look at me like, 'Oh, my God. Look how big I was!' It is an out-of-body experience and they look at themselves like complete aliens. They forget what it is like to be pregnant, which is why it is so important for them to capture that moment."

In Her Own Words:

In Her Pictures

Jennifer, forty, recounts her experience at her pregnancy photo shoot:

"My memories of [the photo shoot] are just as important as the photos themselves. The photographer was really fun and sweet. I told her over the phone that I had body issues but I also wanted to do some partially clothed shots, and the more creative she could be with those, the better. During the shoot, part of which was in my backyard and part of which was in my bedroom, we did several changes of clothing. During my pregnancy I had been too self-conscious to wear a spaghetti tank top, but she encouraged me to wear one [for the photos]. I had also been afraid to wear white because I felt it would make me look even bigger than I was, but she talked me into it. We also found a dress in my closet, which was not a maternity dress but somehow fit me, and it looked great! At one point, she pulled out a newsboy-style cap and put it on me; I never thought I looked good in hats, but I was game. Believe it or not, the photos of me in a white tank and the cap are my favorite photos of myself since my wedding five years ago! During the shoot I just felt beautiful and feminine. By the time we got to the seminude shots in the bedroom, I was comfortable doing whatever she suggested, including laying there in just a pair of underwear. I have to say that in the days that followed, I felt generally more attractive and comfortable with my size (and I wore more tank tops!)."

Ready for Your Close-Up?
Advice for Being Photographed
While Pregnant

Since one of us happens to know a thing or two about modeling, we thought we would pass along a few kernels of wisdom. Follow these tips to get the most out of your photos!

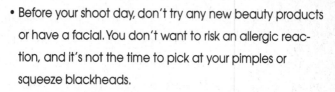

- Before your shoot day, don't try any new beauty products or have a facial. You don't want to risk an allergic reaction, and it's not the time to pick at your pimples or squeeze blackheads.
- Have your favorite music with you, or ready, if you're shooting at your house. Music you love definitely helps get you in a groove, feeling good and in the mood.
- If it's winter, don't wear socks while you're getting ready or going to the studio or you'll have the elastic mark on your legs. Not sexy.
- Bring or have your favorite moisturizer/oil. Before shooting, make sure your skin is glowing, so rub it in.
- If you're in an uncomfortable position while you're posing, it will look uncomfortable in the picture. Speak up and set yourself up to feel good.

Beauty and the Bump

Let this be your mantra throughout your pregnancy: pamper, pamper, pamper! It won't be long before you will be buried in Pampers (you saw that one coming, didn't you?). Take the seats when they're offered, cash in that gift certificate you've been holding onto, and get a prenatal massage. Spend an afternoon or two watching movies in bed. Prop your feet up and read a book cover to cover. Whatever it is that you feel like you never have time to do for yourself, now is your last chance, for the immediate future, at least. We aren't saying that you will never set foot in a spa again, but we won't lie to you—taking care of your newborn will be all-consuming for a while. Treat yourself really well in the months we like to call the calm before the baby poo storm. If you're a low-maintenance girl, move yourself into the medium-maintenance or high-maintenance bracket during pregnancy. Take advantage of all opportunities to lounge and be waited on. This is especially hard for those of us who are used to taking care of everyone else, but you *need* to learn how to take care of yourself before you shift into a role where you will be responsible for taking care of your child unconditionally.

"I've never been one to get manicures or pedicures but have done so a couple of times during pregnancies," said Dede, thirty-two, a mother of two. Treating yourself doesn't have to be in the form of professional treatments, either. It can be as simple as slathering on a mud mask at home and putting a couple of cucumber slices over your eyes. "I'm a pretty low-maintenance person and I don't pay to get a lot of treatments done, but I have found myself taking more time to do my hair, buy nice lotions, take bubble baths, and have my husband give me massages," says twenty-six-year-old Courtney in her thirty-ninth week.

Are All Those Lotions and Potions Safe for Baby?

Pregnancy might make you a little more curious about that long list of ingredients you can't pronounce on your shampoo bottle or moisturizer. Hmmm, what is amyl cinnamal, anyway? If I'm exposing myself to these chemicals, are they safe for my baby?

"I have researched most of the products in my bathroom and makeup cabinet and tossed anything that is considered 'high risk' or unnatural," said Tanya, thirty-seven, in her twenty-eighth week.

Most doctors agree that the majority of makeup and beauty products you can buy in a drugstore are okay to use during pregnancy. However, if switching to all-natural, nontoxic products will help you sleep better at night, by all means go for it. Ask your health care provider about which products are safe and which ones you should avoid.

Manis and Pedis

According to obstetrician Christina Adberg, M.D., the chemicals used in nail salons are only dangerous to you and your baby in extremely high doses (you would pretty much have to be huffing the stuff or spending all day every day in a salon for it to cause any damage). If you do your own nails or get them done professionally while you are pregnant, she recommends staying in a well-ventilated area to minimize your exposure to fumes.

Hair Color

As for those dye jobs, "There have been no human trials that link hair coloring to birth defects," Dr. Adberg says. To be on the safe side, she advises her patients to wait until after the first trimester to color their hair. A knowledgeable stylist should be able to work with you to maintain a look that keeps you feeling confident.

"I have an awful lot of silver hair and I do a lot of 'enhancement.' I wanted to make sure that the dye I was using in my hair wasn't stuff that sits on your scalp," said Erica, thirty-eight. "I talked about it with my stylist. We still did some highlights. If I'd had to give up the coloring completely, that might have thrown me back a little bit."

The drastic physical changes of pregnancy can make you do a double take in the mirror. If indulging in some treatments or painting your nails offsets the shock when you barely recognize your reflection, there's no reason to deny yourself, provided your doctor has given you the thumbs-up. And if you're concerned about your exposure to chemicals or toxic ingredients, there are plenty of alternatives that won't force you to sacrifice your beauty and style.

A Message for Girlfriends! Don't Forget Mommy at the Baby Shower

While you are adding Butt Paste and bibs to your shopping cart, remember to buy a little extra gift just for the mom. Pick up a nice bottle of lotion, bath salts, or a tube of lip gloss—something that your girlfriend didn't add to her registry. She'll be especially appreciative by the end of the party when she's buried in baby onesies.

Safe and Eco-Friendly Beauty and Style

"We live in an overwhelming time. This especially affects new mothers, who have a lot of changes and a lot new information to sort through," says Jessa Blades, an organic beauty consultant and founder of Blades Natural Beauty. "When we are overwhelmed, we tend to jump to extremes—either not caring at all or caring way too much and obsessing." Before you rush out and spend hundreds of dollars on organic products in a panic, Jessa's advice is to prioritize. "Taking small steps, making small changes is so important. Think about what products you use every day. Do you use some of them more than once a day? Start with these products," she advises. The bottom line is that you can begin to make some healthier choices where it matters most, and you don't have to stress yourself out in the process.

Jessa recommends:
   Safe Cosmetics (safecosmetics.org)
   The Cosmetics Database (cosmeticsdatabase.com)

Summer Rayne Oakes, author of *Style, Naturally*, says there are a growing number of designers who are creating eco-friendly fashion for pregnant women and new moms. And you don't need to deck yourself out in a whole new wardrobe of hemp clothing to make a positive impact. "Look for designers who repurpose fabrics and materials. Shopping vintage is also a great way to recycle fashion, instead of adding more products and waste to our world," Summer points out.

Summer's favorites:
   Doie Designs (doiedesigns.com)
   Jessica Scott (jessicascottltd.com)

The Hair Down There

To get the dos and don'ts of preggo bikini maintenance, we turned to Nance Mitchell, a skin care specialist who has waxed some of Hollywoood's biggest stars. Her A-list clients include Gwyneth Paltrow, America Ferrera, and Christina Aguilera.

Nance, who will greet you with a friendly "How's the puss, hon?" if you pay a visit to her Beverly Hills salon, says that it is safe to go for bikini waxes during pregnancy. However, she wasted no time in declaring that it will be a lot more painful than usual because of the increased blood flow to the area. If you do plan to keep yourself tidy and trim while you're pregnant, her advice is to do it regularly.

"You can't start with bushy hair and in your eighth month decide you want to get waxed. It would just be too painful," she warns. Excuse us while we clutch our crotches at the mere idea.

In truth, predelivery waxing is no joke for a lot of women we interviewed. "I was obsessed with the bikini wax during pregnancy!" says Lisa, thirty-five. "I was so worried about what the doctors and nurses would think. Other women, they're more concerned about whether they're going to poop on the table. I didn't care about that. All I cared about was the stupid bikini wax. And I kept asking my husband, 'What do you think? Should I let it grow?' He said, 'No, you should wax it because then they'll be able to see the baby better!'" Nice try, guy. Isn't he aware that all doctors now wear super-powerful goggles that allow them to see through the dark, scary pubic forests so they can deliver every baby safely? Before such innovative technology came along, countless newborns were lost or tangled up in their mothers' over-grown bushes. It was a problem of epidemic proportions, really. Entire civilizations were lost.

We'll Never Tell

Which costar of one of the nineties biggest teen comedies went in for a last-minute bikini wax *while she was in labor*? "She called me at home in the middle of the night and said, 'I'm not going to the hospital looking like this!'" remembers Nance Mitchell. "The doctor was waiting for her and she was in my salon at midnight. She kept telling me, 'Let's just go! Let's do it.' And her doctor was like, 'Where *are* you?'"

Claire says:

"When I saw *Knocked Up*, I let out a shriek during the birth scene—and not because of what they showed. I was more shocked by what was missing. Katherine Heigl (or her vagina stunt double) was 100% Brazilian-style bald! Yikes. As if birth isn't painful enough."

Health care professionals who deliver babies have seen all sorts of fluids and excretions. Let's be honest. They are not likely to be fazed by some pubic hair. But if you prefer to be bare, don't let us stop you.

"Waxing while you're pregnant is actually twice as painful. But I thought, well, it would be a while until I would get to do it again," said Hermione, forty-four, who waxed throughout her pregnancy. For others, it's just an unnecessary hassle. Magali spent a decade of her career being waxed so thoroughly that a stray hair could never be spotted, not even under a magnifying glass. But the dawn of her Hirsute Age directly corresponded with the news that she was pregnant. By delivery day, there was no mist that could conceal the gorilla.

And as far as going back to waxing after delivery? Talk to your doctor about when it is safe. Believe us when we tell you that it will be a while before you want anyone coming near your pubic area with hot wax.

Miracle Stretch-Mark Cream

Oops, there is no such thing. Sorry! But now that we've got your attention, we will take this opportunity to acknowledge that many women we interviewed before and during pregnancy named stretch marks as a top body concern.

We're all for treating yourself to creams, lotions, and oils during pregnancy. Slather them on and let your partner take a turn, too. Just don't get your hopes up that moisturizing your skin will prevent stretch marks. "Unfortunately, whether a mom develops stretch marks or not is often out of her control. The amount of elastin in her skin will help determine if she'll stretch and stay smooth or have stretch marks," says Barbara Dehn, NP, an OB/GYN nurse, and a women's health expert. "Applying creams will keep the skin moist and doesn't hurt, but it probably won't help." And remember, stretch marks do fade over time.

Magali says:

"When I was pregnant, I made my own body oil with about seven differ-ent natural oils I had never heard of before. I stained all my clothes with it because by the end I had no patience to let it dry! But it made me feel special so I didn't mind."

Face Facts

Pregnancy will change your body. You should also be aware that pregnancy hormones might change your face—and we're not talking about "the glow." When you're breaking out like a high school freshman or watching dark blotches appear all over your face, it's hard to feel that you're glowing. In fact, you'll probably feel more like hiding.

Acne

We will spare you the teen magazine advice about not popping pimples (oh, the temptation!) or scrubbing your face raw with a washcloth. On top of those old school no-no's, you can't take acne medication during pregnancy and you need to be extra careful about putting any acne products on your face. Talk to your OB or midwife about safe alternatives. And remember that the hormones making your skin go haywire will settle down after pregnancy.

The Mask of Pregnancy

Hormones can also cause a condition called *chloasma*, which is more commonly known as the mask of pregnancy. Patches of dark skin appear on your face, especially if you have a darker complexion. The sun's UV rays can make the pigment changes even more pronounced, so wear SPF 30 sunblock every day and play "I'm an incognito celebrity in hat and sunglasses" if you're going to be spending time outside. This discoloration usually fades within a few months of delivery, but call your doctor if it persists.

One of the most harmful effects of pregnancy-related skin problems is the damage they do to your self-esteem. If you are isolating yourself from your friends or your partner because you're embarrassed about your appearance, remember that your baby is exposed to that stress and sadness, too. Follow your health care provider's advice, reach out to other women for extra support, and laugh about it if you can. This will not last forever!

What's That Smell?

Prepare for your sense of smell to become extremely sensitive and unpredictable during pregnancy. Do a sniff test on any new products you're considering purchasing to make sure the fragrances don't make you gag. And don't be surprised if your longtime favorite perfume suddenly starts smelling like Eau de Vomit.

If you are especially concerned about the ingredients in your products, eco-expert Summer Rayne Oakes points out that you might want to forgo the perfume entirely during pregnancy in favor of natural oils. "Perfumes are trade secrets, so the companies don't advertise the specific ingredients. You can't read the label and know exactly what's in your perfume," she says.

Checklist: What to Pack for Your Hospital Stay

✓ **Comfy socks.** You don't want to be walking around on the hospital floors in bare feet.

✓ **Flip-flops** for the shower (see above).

✓ **Granny panties in dark colors.** Buy a cheap pack of underwear that you won't mind tossing in the trash after you've worn them. You will experience some serious overflow after giving birth, whether vaginally or by C-section. The last thing you need to worry about is rinsing out your stained panties.

✓ **Ginormous maxipads** (see above).

✓ **Basic toiletries and makeup.** While you probably won't be shaving your legs or plucking your eyebrows in the hospital, you will enjoy a shower after you've had the biggest workout of your life, aka childbirth. Pack your own products so you won't be forced to use the hospital's industrial-grade shampoo and conditioner or wash your face with a sad little bar of standard-issue soap. And if a dab of lip gloss will make you feel human again, by all means bring some. You can count on having at least a few cameras in your face during your stay.

✓ **Roomy clothes to wear home.** By the time you give birth, you will be supremely excited to not be pregnant anymore—an excitement rivaled only by the sheer joy of meeting your little one. But don't delude yourself into thinking that you'll be putting on your prepregnancy jeans to walk out of the hospital. "Nobody mentions that you still look six months pregnant after you give birth!"

says Mara, thirty-five. "When they tell you to pack your bag for the hospital, they say, 'Bring comfortable clothing.' What they don't say is, 'Bring your maternity clothes because your old clothes won't fit you.'" So here we are—telling you to avoid the frustration. Bring some yoga pants or sweats.

Good and Bad Hair Days

Pregnancy Plus: If you've had dreams of becoming a hair model, pregnancy might be the time to go for it. Increased estrogen levels during pregnancy can result in a fuller, thicker head of hair. Try positioning yourself in front of a fan and practice your dramatic slow-motion head tosses.

Postpartum Downer: After childbirth, those estrogen levels will plunge. Good-bye to the luxurious locks and hello to big clumps of hair in the drain! This doesn't happen to all women, but don't freak out if you start shedding. The extreme hair loss is only temporary.

When Can I Build a Bonfire and Toss My Maternity Clothes on It? Style Tips for New Moms

By the end of your pregnancy, you will be beyond sick of your clothing options. The stuff will probably be so stretched out it will be practically transparent. You might also have managed to stain some of it because as you get bigger, your field of vision gets smaller—so you are more likely to bump your bump into random objects and spill things on yourself. Needless to say, you will not be keen to look at any of your maternity outfits once you give birth, let alone actually wear them again. However, you probably won't just fit right back into your prebaby wardrobe. Remember when we told you to pack up all those form-fitting clothes? As tempting as it might be to measure your "progress" by seeing how long it takes you to fit back into them, it's a recipe for torture. Please keep those old clothes under lock and key for a while, and open up another box instead.

Nice Job, Mama! XOXO, Me

Give yourself a gift box to open when you come home from the hospital. Inside:

A beautiful robe and new slippers. Your first weeks home with your new baby will be intense and overwhelming. Your body will be healing and you will be adjusting to a whole new world of responsibilities and routines. If you don't have time to get dressed at first, don't worry about it. Shop for the softest, prettiest robe you can find and get yourself a brand new pair of slippers. You'll be living in them for a little while.

Six-month extras. When you buy tops, yoga pants, and/or leggings to wear around your sixth month of pregnancy, buy a few extras in the same size, but different colors or styles. Don't wear them—don't even cut the tags off. Put them right in your gift box. Instead of stressing about not having anything to wear or not wanting to try on clothes or spend money while you're in between sizes, you'll have a few new, unworn pieces waiting for you.

If You're Planning to Breastfeed . . .

Factor nursing into your shopping decisions. When you look for tops, think about whether they will provide easy access to the boob area. "I try to buy more button-down shirts to be friendly to breastfeeding," says Misty, twenty-nine. Also, keep in mind that breast milk stains. In fact, it stains like nothing else we know of. Even with nursing pads, there will undoubtedly be some accidents, so whites and pastels will quickly get funkified. For this reason (not to mention the spit-up), you'll find darker colors and prints in scale with your body size are a lot more practical.

New Mom, New You

New motherhood is a vulnerable state. You're exhausted and your mind is racing with the "Am I doing this right?" question from minute to minute. As you begin to get a handle on life with your baby, you'll slowly ease into the realm of going out in public. You'll probably start with the basics—taking walks in your neighborhood, going to the grocery store and the doctor's office, then move on to meeting friends, and eventually going back to work (if that's where you're headed).

If you're feeling insecure about your body, getting dressed for any of these outings can be an unpleasant experience, made even more unpleasant by the pressure so many women feel to fight where they are and "go back" to what they were. It's no wonder we feel this way—the "Get your prebaby body back" message is sold to us constantly. But having a child will change your lifestyle, that your goal should be to fit into the sizes and styles you wore before pregnancy. Your style and size choices need to work for your life *now*, not a past-tense version of you.

"I've always had really little breasts and a small stomach. Now I feel like I look like all boob and belly, so I can't wear any of the little tank tops I used to wear," says Sara, a thirty-three-year-old new mom who is having a hard time figuring out how to dress her new body. Before we spoke with her, she admitted that she had just tried on her prepregnancy clothes, and ended up crying on top of a pile of ill-fitting outfits. "It's a whole shift in thinking of what I go for in stores, and what I instantly reach for is no longer what looks good on me. I've had a lot of problems shopping because I can't find things that fit my fashion style and look good on me. You reach for what you know generally looks good on you. Now I have to rethink that."

It can be unsettling to realize that some of the styles you've worn your whole life might not work for you anymore, and some of them might not be practical for every day as they once might have been (OK, maybe they were never "practical," but you didn't really care back then). You don't have to give up wearing heels now that you're a new mom, but it's okay to gravitate toward ballet flats and sneakers more often. After all, stilettos and sandboxes generally don't mix.

It's not that you don't look good in your old clothes. Shift your thinking. It's really your old clothes that don't look good on the new you.

Looking for Affordable Style?

These are some top shopping spots for pregnant women and new moms:

Target (target.com)   Bluefly.com

Zara (zara.com)   Old Navy (oldnavy.com)

H&M (hm.com)   Destination Maternity (destinationmaternity.com)

Beauty Distractions

Instead of agonizing over all the things about your new body you don't like and wish you could change, try experimenting with a new haircut or new makeup. "With my younger two babies, I decided that I wanted to look in the mirror and like what I saw, so I spent a *lot* of time getting my nails and skin cared for," says Sugar, thirty-eight. "I think it was my way of balancing my insecurity about my weight."

Beth, a thirty-three-year-old new mom, tried something she had never tried before: "I'm almost embarrassed to say it. I got fake nails put on! They're horrible for your nails, but I've always been a nail biter and love the look of long, polished nails. So I went to this place near my parents' house and I got French tips put on. Now I will literally sit there and stare at my hands! This is just what makes me feel good about myself. It's really impractical— but so what if I can't pick up my Metrocard when it falls on the ground? I had a little trouble clipping the baby's nails last night because my own nails were in the way, but I just ended up biting her nails, so I still had nails to bite! And if I'm staring at my hands, that means I'm not staring at my stomach and my thighs."

A Message for Girlfriends! Do a Drop-By

Check in on your friend after she's given birth. Reassure her that you don't care if she hasn't made it out of her sweats in a week, and bring her a fun little treat from the beauty aisle instead of a trashy magazine filled with celebrity mommy weight-loss "secrets." She really doesn't need that right now!

"If you have a girlfriend and she's just had a baby, turn up at her house with some nail polish or something (take turns so someone's got dry nails in case you need to pick up the baby)! Being a new mom can be completely isolating and people seem to forget about you altogether. You're left alone and you can't leave the house." —Hermione, 44

Beauty and Style in Its Own Time

Most women are terrified of turning into a "frumpy" mom. But if you took time for your style and beauty before, we are not of the belief that motherhood will turn you into some hideous Hulk-like creature. Yes, you will have to make some adjustments. Your priorities will shift and you'll have to learn how to ask for more help. In the very beginning, you probably will be living in your robe and sweats—and that's okay. Having some frumpy days doesn't mean you are and will forever *be* frumpy.

New You . . .

New shopping habits. You'll probably have less time and less energy to schlep around the stores. If you've never shopped online, give it a try. And when you do venture out, try to stay focused. For the first few times, bring a friend who can provide support and help you maneuver with the baby and all your baby gear.

New curves. Enjoying your new cleavage (not all women do)? Show it off! "I've never had breasts," says Anna, thirty-five. "But now I have them and it's really fun! I've never worn anything with cleavage deeper than my neck and now I keep finding myself in these shirts and dresses and I see people staring at me on the street. 'Yeah, I've got breasts. That's right.'"

New fabrics and colors. When your baby is very small, you'll find yourself going for softer, simple fabrics. Do you really want Junior to get a mouth full of mohair?

Magali says:
"I discovered I was suddenly more interested in bolder, brighter colors when I started shopping for clothes as a mom. If you're feeling more adventurous or you have a taste for something new, go with it!"

New beauty routines. As you enter the world of motherhood, your time for yourself will come in shorter increments and you'll be watching your budget. If you keep an open mind and approach your beauty with a can-do attitude, you'll make the most of the time and money you have. "I do more myself. I do my own pedis, color my own hair, and I have a friend cut it," says Michele, a 36-year-old mother of three.

Return to the style and beauty game in your own time. If you're ready to get dressed up before you're ready to call a babysitter, by all means put on a fancy outfit and order some delivery. Your partner certainly won't complain about seeing you in heels and makeup, even if you're just clacking around your own kitchen for the night. If lack of time forces you to go out in public without the full face you used to put on, and you start to realize that maybe you didn't really need foundation, blush, mascara, eyeliner, eye shadow, and lipstick for a trip to the grocery store anyway—well, we say hurray to that, too.

As your kids get older, things will get easier. But when you're a new mom, having less time, money, and energy does not mean that you are "letting yourself go." Don't make yourself miserable by pining away for all the clothes you used to be able to fit into or putting your style on hold until you've lost all the weight you want to lose. Pack those clothes away (or give some of them away!) and replace them with new items that fit your new shape. Don't mourn all the beauty appointments you used to have time for. Do what you can manage. And remember, sleep is the best beauty treatment of them all.

5

Adding Up, Weighing In, and Counting Down: When All the Numbers Get to Be Too Much

Exactly how much pregnancy weight will I gain?

What will I eat? What will my body look like? How much can I work out when I'm pregnant? How fast will I be able to get back to my size after I give birth? These questions are significant concerns for many women who are accustomed to watching the numbers on the scale. There are plenty of opportunities for mothers and moms-to-be to compare pregnancy pounds and trade stories about weight-loss efforts. That kind of talk is encouraged and those comparisons are nearly impossible to avoid. But beneath all the talk about extra flab and stretch marks are more serious worries—worries that aren't such acceptable topics of conversation. Will I be a good enough mother? Will I lose control of all the routines that have been so central to my life? Will I resent my child for "ruining" my body? What do I say when I don't feel as happy and excited as everyone expects me to be? Our weight chatter often masks deep silences and carefully guarded secrets.

Julia, a thirty-six-year-old mother of two who suffered from bulimia as a teenager and now considers herself recovered, admits that she keeps her history close to the vest. "When I talk to my girlfriends about someone being too skinny, I never bring my personal history into the conversation. I keep that out completely. It's not something I talk about now. It's not something I want people around me to know I had, only because it has such a negative connotation. People think, 'Oh, yeah. Another girl who was puking.'"

No one likes to be labeled. But the truth is that there *are* a lot of us puking girls and starving girls out there. Until we got help and did a lot of work to get ourselves healthy, we were two of them. The National Eating Disorders Association estimates that 10 million women in the United States suffer from eating disorders, such as anorexia and bulimia, and millions more are struggling with binge-eating disorder. These are complex illnesses with complex roots, ranging from the biological to the cultural.

It took a long time to name our behavior and own our past experiences. It's been an ongoing process that has come with plenty of triumphs and setbacks. Sure, sometimes it does seem easier to keep quiet and avoid judgment, especially when so many people have such misconceptions about eating disorders. But for us, sweeping our histories under the rug only serves to reinforce the stigma so many women feel. As women, as mothers, and as future mothers, none of us should have to hide in shame.

Shapes of Gray: What Is Disordered Eating?

In addition to the huge number of women who have or once had full-blown eating disorders, a 2008 University of North Carolina/*Self* magazine study found that 65 percent of all American women are disordered eaters. In other words, more than two-thirds of us have some issues in the food and weight department.

"There are behaviors that fall under the radar," says Cynthia Bulik, Ph.D., director of the University of North Carolina Eating Disorders Program. "With disordered eating, you don't necessarily meet the diagnostic criteria for anorexia, bulimia, or binge-eating disorder, but you have pieces of any of those that cause you distress or interfere with your life and well-being."

It is often hard to recognize when your behavior is disordered because these damaging attitudes about food and weight have become so "normal" in our day-to-day lives. We see them all around us—in our families, in our offices, among our friends. We looked at six categories of disordered eating* and we found that many of the women we surveyed and interviewed fell into one or several of them. If you recognize yourself in any of these descriptions, take our word for it that freeing yourself from these

*Categories outlined by Self magazine and the University of North Carolina at Chapel Hill in their 2008 study (published in the May 2008 issue).

behaviors will be the best thing you ever do for yourself. We encourage you to reach out for help if you haven't already. Not only is disordered eating harmful and stressful, it can impact your pregnancy and your ability to pass along healthy habits to your children.

Calorie Prisoners

❏ Are you petrified of gaining weight? Do you scrutinize food labels, know how many calories are in all your meals, and count them up all day? Do you think of food in terms of "bad" or "good" and feel guilty if you stray?

Secret Eaters

❏ Do you eat junk food in private? Do you snack in your car or at home when you won't be found out?

Career Dieters

❏ Do you feel lost without a diet plan? Have you tried every fad diet in the book and still feel as if your weight is out of control? Many women who are overweight or obese fall into this category.

Food Addicts

❏ Do you eat to deal with emotions like stress and anger? Do you seek comfort in food or find yourself thinking about food all the time?

Purgers

❏ Do you resort to using laxatives, diuretics, or occasional vomiting to get rid of unwanted calories?

Extreme Exercisers

❏ Do you feel anxious or upset if you have to miss a workout? Do you push yourself to exercise even when you are injured or sick?

Voices of Disordered Eating

"I have the usual stories about crying after accidentally drinking regular Coke, refusing to eat food I hadn't made myself, etc."

—Alicia, 28, who plans to have children

"Now that I am pregnant, I look back and realize that I was in great shape before my pregnancy . . . I struggle to eat healthy most of the time and find that I am hard on myself (very critical) when I eat 'bad foods.'"

—Lori, 34, who is 21 weeks pregnant

"I think I have the type of disordered eating many women have: feeling guilty about eating things, counting calories, occasionally binge-ing, then feeling bad. My parents are very strict about eating and weight, so I used to snack in secret. [I am] learning more about body issues . . . and I am starting to try to think differently about myself."

—Natalie, 23, who does not plan to have children

"I have dieted on and off from childhood until age 30. I am considered clinically 'obese.'"

—Lena, 31, who plans to have children

"I chose to crash-diet in high school. I also started fasting . . . until I started fainting. The consensus [from my doctors during my pregnancy] was that I was overweight because I had screwed up

my metabolism with ridiculous dieting techniques, and that
pregnancy was a chance to reset my metabolism."   —Sara, 31, mother

"I can be a bit of an emotional eater. If I feel sad or lonely or empty on
the inside, sometimes I eat."   —Candace, 24, who plans to have children

"I'm an emotional eater who has often slid into terrible bouts of binge
eating. And I do have a rather poor body image, which of course fuels
the emotional eating. [Sigh]"   —Amanda, 35, mother

"I am constantly striving to be thin and have suffered from all sorts
of eating disorders, never getting serious but on the verge thereof. I
now have come to terms that even if I hit my dream weight, I still
won't be happy. I have used laxatives. Also I have also thrown up,
more so spit up, several times and still have trouble with that."
                                        —Sheena, 23, who plans to have children

"I have almost always hated my body. The times when I have felt
most beautiful, I was usually starving or sacrificing loads of time to
exercise."   —Misty, 30

"[Now] I will miss a workout for a sick child, and many other rea-
sons. Before children, there was no reason that would make me miss a
workout. I used to work out every day."   —Michelle, 40, mother

"I've never stopped eating, but my body image is always *on my mind!*
When I was 17 to 18 years old, I went to the gym every day just to
keep thin."   —Elin, 26, who plans to have children

Some women get officially diagnosed with eating disorders and many, many others live in that disordered gray area, over-working their muscles on treadmills, overworking their digestive systems on diet after diet, or overworking their tear ducts in front of full-length mirrors. We are set up to believe that as long as we're not "dying to be thin" (insert ominous voiceover and shot of an emaciated teen girl picking forlornly at the food on her plate), we're okay. It's those other women who have the real problems. If we purge once a month, we're confident that we're better off than someone who's purging once a week. If we eat uncontrollably once a week? Well, at least it's not a daily thing. If we cancel plans because we feel too guilty about skipping a workout, we're just trying to get in shape. And if we weigh our-selves religiously twice a day, what's wrong with taking charge of our health? We run these justifications through our heads until we convince ourselves that they are true, but rarely do we utter them out loud, and when we do, those around us are quick to respond with their own body bashing. Instead of, "Come on, what's really bothering you," we get "You think your thighs are fat? Check out these wobbly arms!" Instead of reaching out for help, we talk about pounds and calories. These conversations are even more damaging when we become mothers. We get valida-tion of our unhealthy behavior, and we risk passing our body-obsessed language on to our children.

What's Eating Us? The Heavy Burden
of Keeping Our Weight Fears Under Wraps

If millions of women suffer from diagnosable eating disorders and millions more are disordered eaters, it doesn't take a rocket scientist to figure out that a sizable percentage of those women are or will someday become mothers. But even though pregnancy and motherhood are arguably the most body-transforming and life-transforming experiences a woman will go through, there is not a whole lot of support for the countless moms and moms-to-be who struggle with food, weight, and body-image problems. As soon as we pee on that stick and it reveals a plus sign, we're expected to be 100-percent focused on the baby's health and ready to pack on the pounds—immediately setting aside the weight worries that came before. Meanwhile, women's magazine headlines continue to preach about how to find "the thinner, happier you!" and every tabloid and entertainment Web site runs incessant stories about postbaby weight loss and celebrity mom slim-down secrets. But we're not supposed to talk about how crippling our weight-gain fears can be. Pregnant women beat themselves up for not having the perfect-sized bump, and then they feel guilty for worrying about such silliness. New mothers torture themselves by trying on their prebaby skinny jeans, and then they feel guilty when they can't resist comparing their bodies to those of the other moms at the park.

Even young women with no immediate plans to have children tread cautiously when they approach the topic of body image, pregnancy, and motherhood. "Motherhood is seen as this great,

heavenly experience," confesses nineteen-year-old Linda. "Address-
ing any downsides beyond labor pains would be practically blas-
phemous." Twenty-one-year old Marie says that she and her
friends are already talking out the body changes they will face
when they eventually h children, but she is careful not to
reveal too much. "We al e that we are scared to gain weight,
but I don't let them k now deep my fear really is." Jenny,
twenty-five, was dia d with anorexia at the age of fifteen.
"Even though my g friends is incredibly close and we talk
about everything dy image is the one issue that never
seems to come u ys. "It's almost like it's too sensitive and
we're afraid to or set someone off. We all maintain the
'Oh, I eat wh I want and would never let society tell me
how to feel yself' illusion with each other, though I doubt
we are all that strong all the time." Jenny has recovered
from her disorder and wants to have children in the future,
but she ave some reservations. "I've reached the point
where tand my body—what it can and can't do, what it
need healthy, etc. I fear changes that I can't predict or
con d having to repeat the process of getting to know
m this way. I feel terribly selfish even thinking that and I
 ink it would *stop* me from having kids, but upsetting my
on balance of confidence in my body is scary."

elfish is a word that gets thrown around a lot when women
lk about motherhood. It is a dreaded slur among mommies and
nommies-to-be who are sure they will get slapped with the label
if they admit how concerned they really are about pregnancy
weight gain and postbaby weight loss. Sadly, their fears are not

entirely unfounded. Vicki Iovine, author of the bestselling *The Girlfriends' Guide to Pregnancy*, takes a major detour from her otherwise empathetic advice to hurl some choice words at anyone who dares to let her food and weight issues affect her pregnancy.

[I]t should be understood that the baby's health is more important than any other consideration, and that any woman who starves herself or eats only trash foods should permanently be ostracized from the community of Girlfriends, if not from the universe.

Ouch. Of *course* it's dangerous for a woman to starve herself or binge on junk food throughout her pregnancy. You won't find too many people who will argue with that. The irony is that for women to get those issues in check, we have to be able to talk about them first. We need to know that we won't be chastised. We must feel safe enough to ask for help. Telling moms-to-be that they'll be booted off the island and friendless forever if they let their body worries—and the deeper insecurities that drive them— out of the closet is not exactly the best way to create a circle of trust now, is it?

That brand of put-down is nothing new. It's existed for generations, in fact, even turning up in *Mad Men*, the hit TV show depicting the advertising world of the early 1960s. In one episode, the character of Betty Draper purses her painted red lips as her doctor informs her that she is pregnant. Betty has just learned that her husband is cheating on her. She's depressed, confused, and in the midst of an identity crisis of *Feminine Mystique* proportions. "Are you sure?" she asks her doctor. He reads the fear on her face. "Are you concerned about your appearance?" he responds, with eyebrows raised. "You've been blessed with a very resilient figure." It is at once a total brush-off of her real problems and a reinforcement of a mixed message that is still going strong today: We ladies are *expected* to devote ourselves to maintaining, improving, and talking about our figures, but we had better not get too carried away with it. Why? Well, because it's just so "silly."

Under the threat of such harsh judgment, it's not surprising that women work so hard to carefully guard the seriousness of their food and weight obsessions. For mothers and women who are pregnant, the pressure to maintain that image of togetherness is ever-present. Sara, a thirty-three-year-old new mom, had been planning to lose weight when she found out she was pregnant. She ditched the diet plans for nine months but admits that she started thinking about weight loss again the day after she gave birth. She restricted her meals to just fish, salads, yogurt, and fruit during the first two weeks of her daughter's life, until she realized that cutting her calorie intake so drastically wasn't healthy for her breastfeeding baby. Now when she goes out to eat with her friends, she gets self-conscious when everyone else is ordering appetizers for their main course and she wants something more substantial. "I feel like I'm the heaviest in the group now, so I should really watch what I'm eating," she says. "It's ridiculous. I would consider myself smart and educated. Intellectually, I know if I were to talk to anyone about body image or nutrition, they would say to me that I look exactly the way I'm supposed to look for having had a baby twelve weeks ago. I'm doing all the things I'm supposed to be doing. I'm eating relatively healthy. But I can't help it that every time I look in the mirror, I think, 'Oh, I look disgusting.' I feel almost ashamed about not liking the way I look. So I've chosen not to tell people about it."

Carla, thirty-five, has struggled with bouts of bulimia since she was nineteen. While she no longer throws up several times a day, as she did when she was in college, she still has occasional relapses. She told us she purged twice while she was pregnant and now she sometimes binges and purges when her husband is away on business trips—a secret she had told no one.

"When I'm sitting home alone and I'm having one of those days and I see all these little yummy mummies prancing down the road with their Bugaboo strollers and their Seven jeans and Lulu Guinness sweaters, it's just like, 'Holy fucking pass the pie!' And then you eat the pie and the corn chips and the pasta and pretty much everything else you can find in the house during the baby's nap. And then you look again at all the skinny mommies and you look at yourself and your baby is five-and-a-half months old and you still can't fit into your fat pants—and you head for the sink with the teaspoon," she admits.

"I'm supposed to be above all that, right? I'm supposed to know that if I don't feel pretty, it's because of unrealistic stereotypes of women," says Carla. "Look, I know all about unrealistic stereotypes and how mass-produced media makes us feel like crap. But I still *feel* like crap."

Sadly, at those times when what we know fails to match what we feel as we stand in front of the mirror, we don't open up and reach out—we shut up and close off. We don't talk about what's eating away at us; we talk about what we should and shouldn't be eating.

Scam Alert: The "Perfect" Body

Pregnancy and first-time motherhood come with heaping doses of self-doubt. Sure, being preggers and becoming a mom change your body. However, let's not forget that they also turn the rest of your world topsy-turvy. There can be joyful, blissed-out highs, but also plenty of moments when that nasty voice creeps inside your head to ask, "What the hell did I do? Who told me this would be a good idea?" And what do we do when we start freaking out that we're not good enough, smart enough, or together enough to handle the mommy gig? Well, it's not long before we start questioning everything else in our lives, and measuring our waistlines to determine if we're thin enough and pretty enough, too.

The allure of the Perfect Body is hardest to resist when life seems out of control (like, you know, when your kid's got a raging diaper rash or when the new mom listserv you joined starts clogging your inbox with diatribes proclaiming the evils of the nonorganic baby food you just bought twenty jars of). The Perfect Body promises to melt away all those nagging insecurities, replacing them with a flat, toned stomach and smooth legs devoid of anything remotely resembling cottage cheese. It is the magic self-esteem elixir sought by women far and wide. Except there's one small problem. Try as you might, it is impossible to reach. You can gain just the right amount of weight during pregnancy, but that doesn't mean you won't get some stretch marks. You can shed ten pounds of that baby weight you've been trying to lose, but suddenly fifteen seems like a better goal. You can work out three times a week, but then you start thinking that things won't truly fall into place until you can somehow manage five.

Our years of disordered eating have taught us that the never-ending quest for the Perfect Body is one giant scam. It's equivalent to a late-night infomercial that somehow convinces you that your life will be transformed if you act now and order a towel that can soak up Lake Michigan in ten minutes, or a clip-on light that will help you excavate the depths of your purse. Feeling stressed, depressed, inferior, or inadequate? Weight loss is presented as the magic solution. But, in reality, it only provides a temporary thrill, like when that little light shines on a forgotten treasure clinging to the lining of your bag. Your first step to total life organization? No, wait. It's just a crusty, hairy peppermint that's probably old enough to be your kid's babysitter.

Body image and eating disorders therapist Lesley Goth, PsyD, likens this disappointment setup to a mousetrap—and the unrelenting photo barrage of celebrity new moms makes for perfect bait. "I've had patients obsess over these pictures of stars in the spotlight who have just had babies. It's right in their faces every day and there is this perpetual cycle of frustration that they can't attain those goals," she says. But if your big-picture goals are health and happiness, Goth points out that at the end of the day it's not the chefs, personal trainers, or nannies you really need. "The pressure to lose the weight is like a cover-up for much deeper issues. If women can really stop and think—talk to a friend, talk to a pastor or a rabbi or a counselor, or get into some kind of support group—they can really start to look at what's going on underneath so they don't have to fall into this trap."

Doctors: They Don't Ask, We Don't Tell

There is a tremendous amount of shame surrounding eating disorders, disordered eating, and serious body-image issues. It is hard enough to be honest about our experiences with our friends and partners, and even harder to open up to our doctors. Obstetricians, midwives, and other health care professionals rarely get the full story about their patients' eating disorder histories or body-image concerns.

Dangerous Silences

- Of those we surveyed, 73 percent of pregnant women with body-image issues and histories of eating disorders and disordered eating said they have not discussed this history with their obstetrician or midwife.
- Seventy-nine percent of mothers with body-image issues and histories of eating disorders and disordered eating said they did not discuss this history with their obstetrician or midwife.

Lucy, thirty-seven, has dealt with a distorted body image for most of her life, but she hasn't raised these issues with her obstetrician. "I'm worried that I'll get the typical response of, 'That's normal. You're not overweight. Don't worry about it.'" she explains. Lori, thirty-four, has what she describes as a "tumultuous" relationship with food and her body image. At week twenty-one of her pregnancy, she's nervous about how much total weight she'll gain and that she won't be able to lose it or get back in shape after giving birth. "I keep it to myself, because most people don't truly understand the concerns," she says. "I don't feel that medical practitioners today are really open to hearing the details of eating issues or body-image issues."

Lucy and Lori aren't off base. Again and again, we've heard stories of doctors who have been completely clueless and sometimes downright insensitive to the weight triggers and land mines that so many women face during pregnancy and as new mothers. Cynthia Bulik, Ph.D. works to educate obstetricians and their nurses about how to more effectively treat women with eating disorders and body-image issues. She is quick to acknowledge that there is a lot of progress yet to be made. "They throw you on the scale, they don't even look at you, and with their paper and pencil in hand, they weigh you," she says. "I've had so many moms with eating disorders say things like, 'I didn't eat for two days before my appointment because I didn't want them to see how much weight I had gained.' It's really scary when your visit to your doctor is so uncomfortable that you feel like you have to restrict." Clearly, that kind of behavior is not healthy for the baby. But it's not healthy for the *mother*, either. And it's the mother's health and emotional well-being that often gets lost in the mix of weight charts and scales.

Obstetricians and midwives aren't psychologists; they shouldn't be expected to diagnose and treat eating disorders, but they *should* know that statistics show that a good number of their patients will have some form of disordered eating in their past or present and that pregnancy is a sensitive time for women who struggle with these issues. Amanda, a thirty-year-old mother of two, has a history of anorexia. Her primary care doctor was aware of this history, and because her obstetrician's office uses the same computerized documentation system and had access to all her medical records, she assumed that her prenatal care providers were aware, too. "I thought it might come up because with both my pregnancies I had a difficult time gaining weight," she told us. "Between both my pregnancies I saw seven different obstetricians and two midwives because it was recommended to have an appointment with each person in the practice, and not one of them ever mentioned anything." It should be noted that Amanda didn't mention anything, either. She is in the majority. Most women don't bring up the issue; most doctors never ask.

Those who do find the courage to broach the subject with their doctors are too often met with exactly the judgmental or dismissive attitudes that prevent others from speaking up.

Niki, twenty-five, has suffered with bulimia, compulsive binge eating, and obsessive thoughts about her body. Sixteen weeks pregnant, she describes herself as "gross, swollen, and fat." Her doctor was none too pleased to hear that Niki was feeling anxious about the pregnancy weight gain. "She looked at me kind of upset and said, 'You do realize you have to eat?' She is only concerned about the baby but doesn't seem to realize that I am, too. And I am trying to be healthy, just like anyone," Niki says.

Julia, thirty-six, went to her doctor to discuss an unplanned pregnancy and was reprimanded for expressing her fears: "I went in there completely scared and neurotic and I felt like she just

wanted me out that door. I switched doctors after that because
. . . she was aware of my history with an eating disorder and did
not do anything to help me calm down. Maybe she thought she
was just going to give me tough love and tell it like it is and say,
'You're going to get fat. Deal with it.' That was not working for
me. She didn't have any sympathy for my situation."

It's these strained interactions that stand in the way of women
getting the care and support they need to deal with the body
changes of pregnancy. In an ideal world, every obstetrician and
midwife would be well-equipped to recognize the signs when one
patient breaks out in a cold sweat at the prospect of stepping on
the scale, or another one seems especially persistent when inquiring about whether her weight gain is "normal." Instead of the typical "Calm down" or "You really have to start thinking of the
baby's health," we might start hearing about doctors who tell their
patients that there's no shame in seeking help for disordered eating and who give referrals to qualified therapists. Unfortunately,
short of requiring every prenatal care provider to go through sensitivity training, there is no way to guarantee that utopian scenario. But the more upfront we are as patients, the better our
chances of finding health care providers who won't brush us off
or shame us into silence.

Dr. Christina Adberg, an obstetrician who practices in Beverly
Hills (an area that takes the term *body conscious* to a whole new
level), advises women to be proactive in discussing their body-
image concerns and eating disorder histories with their OBs or
midwives. "I talk a lot about diet as part of my intake. Sometimes
a patient's worries will come out as a part of that conversation,

like, 'Oh, I don't want to think that much about my weight. I don't want to know how much I weigh—don't tell me how much I weigh.' And then the lightbulb goes off for me."

Dr. Adberg says that she will weigh a patient backwards and not reveal the number if there is any danger that it might become an unhealthy fixation. Yes, you read that right. This might seem radical in light of the fact that the scale has become the looming centerpiece of most OB checkups, but in most cases, there is absolutely no medical reason for a woman to know her specific weight throughout pregnancy. "I'll only discuss their weight with them if it's a problem," Dr. Adberg explains. "I generally don't walk in the door and look at their weight on the chart and say, 'Oh, we've got to talk about your weight.' I'm not one of those doctors who lectures people. There is so much variation, so if the baby is measuring right and they are the same person I remember seeing a month ago, then I'm not freaking out about it." Dr. Adberg recommends that patients remind the nurse of their preference not to be told their weight at the beginning of each checkup.

Sandra, a thirty-two-year-old mother of two who suffered from bulimia for fifteen years, says her midwife did not even weigh her past her first trimester. "She would measure me and do my glucose test. In the end, I truly do not know how much I gained because I did not even get on a scale at home!" she remembers.

Finding a doctor or midwife with a nonjudgmental outlook and some body-image savvy is important, especially for women who are nervous about eating disorder-related health complications or whether pregnancy itself could trigger disordered eating or severe anxieties about weight. Consider your search for a health care provider like an interview—you're on the hiring end. The best way to gauge what kind of doctor you're dealing with is to push through whatever shame or guilt you might be feeling and put your issues—whether they are in your distant past or you're dealing with them on a daily basis—on the table right away. If you're met with criticism or any other reaction that makes you uncomfortable, remember that you are well within your rights to say, "Thanks, but no thanks" and walk right out that door. People have a tendency to cower and bow to doctors, to our own detriment. When they are disrespectful, we assume we must have done something to deserve the attitude. When they are condescending, we blame ourselves for being too stupid or naive. This self-flagellating tendency is especially prevalent among women with food and weight issues. For our health and the health of our children, we need to get over it and muster every ounce of bad-ass we've got when we're choosing the health care providers who are going to help us bring our babies into the world. We do not, under any circumstances, deserve to be belittled or berated for having the courage to be honest.

Magali says:

"After seven years of suffering with bulimia and letting my weight determine how I felt about myself from minute to minute, I threw out my scale as part of my recovery and haven't owned one since. When I got pregnant, I started seeing an obstetrician who couldn't quite get his head around the fact that I didn't want to know my weight. He flat-out ignored my request and every time I went in for an appointment, my weight was the first thing that was recited to me. So I had to give him the proverbial boot, and I found a midwife with better listening skills. It's amazing what happens when you take weight out of the pregnancy equation. For one thing, you start to realize how much those numbers typically dominate women's conversations. Girlfriends (or other random strangers, for that matter) would ask how much weight I had gained at various points in the pregnancy, and it was quite freeing to be able to respond honestly, "I have no idea." It was as if I had told them I was planning to take up residence on the moon or something. They would get this disoriented look on their faces, like they couldn't figure out what else we could possibly talk about. But once people get past the initial shock that you're not up for trading notes about weight, you'll start to discover that there are endless other topics to discuss—topics that are a whole lot more interesting than pounds and ounces."

In addition to the fear of being shamed or shut down, many women told us they don't bring up their eating-disorder histories or body-image issues with their obstetricians or midwives because it was all just so long ago it doesn't seem relevant anymore. "I did not really discuss my poor body image with my midwife. I felt I had mostly made peace with it enough so that it was not really an issue that would interfere with my giving birth," explained thirty-six-year-old Karen. Tara, twenty-nine, who suffered with eating disorders earlier in her life, said simply, "I was well over all this by the time I became pregnant."

As two women who have been free from our eating disorders for well over a decade, we understand how those days of bingeing, purging, and meticulously tracking every freaking calorie and fat gram that touched our lips can seem like ancient history, a past life even. For those of us who consider ourselves recovered (or at least on the healthy side of recovery), it's a strange trip to revisit those times. Prolonged self-starvation, excessive exercise, vomiting, laxative abuse, yo-yo dieting, compulsive eating—whatever your drug of choice, they all cloud the memory. Those days are hazy, so dark, private, and surreal that it can seem almost impossible to articulate what went on. Do you really have to unearth all that ugliness now? The short answer is yes. If you want to be the healthiest mom you can be, you do need to acknowledge that these issues and illnesses have shaped you. Whether they are part of your past or present, the truth is that pregnancy and motherhood can tap into some of the very vulnerabilities that are at the root of eating disorders and food and weight obsessions. This is not to say that every woman who has suffered with an eating disorder or felt bad about her body will necessarily have to confront those demons during pregnancy, after childbirth, or as a mother. Some women find that pregnancy and motherhood liberate them from their disordered eating and food and weight issues. Others find themselves turning to unhealthy behaviors as a way of coping with the tidal wave of emotions that come with these experiences. Until you are in the thick of it, so to speak, there is no surefire way to predict how you will be affected. That's why we think all women should go into pregnancy with an awareness of the possible triggers and how to deal with them.

Be on the Lookout:
Triggers of Pregnancy and New Motherhood

Disclaimer: This is a "Heads-up, ladies. You're not the only one" list, *not* to be confused with a "Holy crap, you're totally screwed" list. Familiarize yourself with these triggers so you can be prepared to reach out for help should one or any combination of these interconnected issues start hitting too close to home.

Control (or Total Lack of It)

There's just not a heck of a lot we get to control about pregnancy and new motherhood. "Being a new mom, there is so much insecurity about whether you're going to be good at it. There's so much fear, which feels out of control. That can trigger eating-disordered behavior and the need to go out of your way to control everything and everyone," warns eating disorders therapist Lesley Goth, PsyD.

Miscarriage

About 15 to 20 percent of all known pregnancies end in miscarriage. The loss is profound, and women who experience miscarriage often feel as though their bodies betrayed them. "If there's a miscarriage or if anything else goes wrong in the pregnancy, that can lead to self-blame that can trigger the need to self-punish," says Lesley Goth, PsyD.

Miscarriage is a hush-hush topic in our culture, which can make it even harder for women to seek support when they need it most. "In the first three months of your pregnancy you're discouraged from telling anybody because of this whole idea that if you have a miscarriage, it's some kind of shameful thing," says Amy, thirty-seven. "Granted, it's a personal issue, but that's a real grief women go through and I don't understand why you're supposed to be so secretive. If I lose the baby it's like it didn't exist?"

Superwoman Syndrome

Many women who have suffered with eating disorders are also perfectionists. Get ready for the Perfect Mommy pressure cooker. "Women believe that we have to be superwomen all the time. We have to work when we are eight months pregnant and still go to the gym. I think everyone wants to be perfect and if you're not perfect, then you feel like you are weak," says Kristen, a thirty-four-year-old mother of three with a history of bulimia who did not binge and purge during pregnancy, but she did find herself very susceptible to the perfection triggers. "Everyone asks, 'How much did you gain? Did you have a C-section or deliver vaginally? Are you going to baby yoga? Are you doing it all?' My pregnancies were tough, so I wasn't doing it all. It was easier to say, 'Everything is fine.' I was lying, but it was just easier to not get into it." Which brings us right to our next trigger. . . .

Alone in "the Glow"

Awaiting the arrival of your baby is a time of anticipation and excitement. But what if, despite all the buzz of planning and preparation, you aren't the over-the-moon-happy pregnant woman everyone expects you to be? Bringing your baby home is the moment you've been waiting for, isn't it? But how do you explain yourself when you feel desperately lonely and disconnected from

the blissful experience you're "supposed" to be having? Your
friends assume that you're swamped and don't call, and there you
are, *alone* in the house wiping your baby's ass and trying to come
to grips with the stark realization that your life is forever changed
and you're facing so many unknowns. You can expect emotional
ups and downs, but be careful not to close up or isolate yourself
when you're experiencing them. Women with eating-disorder histories are experts at putting on our outside happy faces and then
locking ourselves inside to numb our loneliness with the rituals
we don't talk about. "When I had the little one, the first few
months were an absolute nightmare," says Carla, thirty-five, who
found herself bingeing during the many hours she spent on her
own with her newborn. "I was isolated a lot. Especially since I
was breastfeeding. I was just trapped. And breastfeeding does
make you really, really hungry."

The Mother of All Issues

When you become a mom, it's only natural to do some serious reflecting on your relationship with *your* mom, and maybe
your dad, and whoever else had a part in raising you—for better or worse. "It brings up your childhood. You start thinking
about all the things you want to do or not do differently from
your own mom," says Dr. Goth. We both grew up with loving,
supportive parents and we both ended up with eating disorders.
There isn't always a "bad mommy" to blame, but family dynam-
ics can certainly play a role in how we deal with food and
weight. Recovering from an eating disorder requires us to understand, from a daughter's perspective, how the words and actions

of our parents affected us. As a mother-to-be, there's a new world of responsibility on your plate. How will *your* words and actions affect your children? We told you this stuff was heavy.

Deep Wounds

Pregnancy and new motherhood can sometimes bring up memories of past trauma. "If there has been past abuse or molestation, which is very common with people who have eating disorders, being pregnant could trigger memories of that abuse," says Lesley Goth, PsyD. She also says that some women are triggered by memories of past abortions or children they gave up for adoption: "Even if the decisions were good decisions at the time, it could still trigger guilt and shame during the pregnancy and after childbirth."

Bingeing for Two

While research shows that many women with eating disorders like anorexia and bulimia go into remission during pregnancy, a recent University of North Carolina study revealed an unexpected increase in new cases of binge-eating disorder that actually *began* in pregnancy. To be clear, bingeing isn't just a response to increased hunger. It's what happens when the emptiness we feel inside just doesn't seem to disappear, no matter how much food we consume. "For some women, especially those who lacked the support to deal with the stress of pregnancy, it ended up being a triggering time period rather than a reprieve from binge eating," says Cynthia Bulik, Ph.D. One explanation could be that bingeing during pregnancy doesn't come with the same social stigma that self-starvation and purging do. Bulik compares purging to smoking during pregnancy—it's the kind of behavior that sets off alarms that you're doing something that could really harm your baby. Eating uncontrollably, on the other hand, fits right into the "Go ahead, you're eating for two" pregnancy mythology; heck, it's practically socially acceptable. But that doesn't mean it's healthy. "Nutrients in utero are really important. What we're concerned about with all these binge-eating disorder cases is that the babies are getting really erratic exposure to large quantities of food. That can potentially negatively affect their growth and health trajectory," she warns.

If years of carefully counting and cutting calories have messed with your ability to trust your own appetite and eat intuitively, it's not a stretch to see how the "Give in to your pregnancy cravings" green light immediately followed by the "Lose your baby weight *now!*" siren can spell trouble. Bulik notes that, in her experience, women who go for quantity over quality in their pregnancy food choices are more likely to be shell-shocked by their weight gain later. "Those are the women who get really freaked because they gained more weight than they wanted to," she says. "What they've told me is that they're really worried about it, and they feel like once the baby's out they have no more 'excuses.' Sometimes they won't even eat enough to sustain breastfeeding. They want to lose baby weight as fast as they can. And that puts a huge stress on their bodies and their minds."

Did You Know?

According to a 2008 study conducted by the University of North Carolina, women who tried to restrict their diets in some way before pregnancy gained more weight during pregnancy than women who were not dieters.

Another 2008 study, conducted by researchers at Harvard Medical School and Harvard Pilgrim Health Care, showed that normal-weight women who thought they weighed more than they actually did had *twice the odds of gaining excessive weight* during their pregnancy.

The Weighting Game

Counting, weighing, comparing, measuring—these are all familiar eating-disorder rituals. And then comes pregnancy, with its seemingly endless opportunities to—yep, you guessed it—count, weigh, compare, and measure. Kim, thirty-two, was bulimic in college. When she became pregnant with her first child at twenty-eight, she worried about gaining too much weight. "As with the bulimia, I tried to keep a mental note of what I was eating and keep it in check. I wrote everything down. I tracked my calories and tracked how much I gained each trimester to make sure I would not go over what the doctor recommended," she remembers. It might feel as if you're in control when you're stringently watching calorie intake and weight gain during and after pregnancy, but it's more likely that your obsessive thoughts about food and weight are controlling you. If your efforts to stay exactly in the weight range your doctor recommends make it impossible for you to relax or think about much else, the emotional stress you're putting yourself through might just be canceling out the health benefits of maintaining your "perfect" pregnancy weight.

How Will Pregnancy Affect Me?

"I am worried that I won't be able to 'take a vacation' from obsessing over my weight during this period of time to take care of the baby. I've struggled with anorexia for eight years. I don't talk openly about the eating disorder or body image in general. Additional concerns of mine are the ability to have children (due to infertility issues caused by the eating disorder) and passing the eating disorder on to my children since there is a high genetic component."

—Katie, 24, who wants to have children

"I have struggled with anorexia and binge-eating disorder (switching between the two) on and off for about eight years. I am terrified of gaining the weight, even though I know I will need to for the health of my baby. I am scared that I won't be able to enjoy having my child growing and developing inside of me because I will feel like a huge fat cow. I am afraid that after I have the baby . . . I won't be able to lose the weight fast enough for my own standards."

—Sarah, 24, who wants to have children

"I'm worried that I won't let myself gain the necessary weight, and even more worried that I won't lose it afterwards—although I've always been thin, I'll be revealed as the 'fat girl' I always should have been. Having considered it, it is absolutely my fear. It's ironic—we're talking about creating a family, producing a life, and all I can think about is my pants size. Perhaps not ironic, just sad."

—Denise, 31, who describes herself as "anorexic-ish" since age 17, and plans to have children

"I've been triggered so many times—big triggers—while in recovery. I'm just not sure that I could handle (A) pregnancy weight gain, (B) some serious lack of control over what's happening to my body, (C) the reality of having to be responsible for a child when I'm scared I'll never be through with my own issues. I'd likely adopt if I were to decide to raise a child."

—Libby, 31

"My hunch is that, if [I were] pregnant, I would become more in tune with my body, and it would be a beneficial experience. However, I wonder how I would deal with the extra weight after or the permanent changes in my body, not to mention the amount of focus that would have to be taken off myself to care for a child. I want to become more in touch with my body and moods. I'm certainly not ready for children yet, but I hope to one day feel ready for the challenge/growth. It's definitely a huge unknown. I also feel very passionately that I do not want to pass on any eating disorder behavior to a child."

—Michelle, 26, in recovery from anorexia, binge-eating disorder, and compulsive exercise

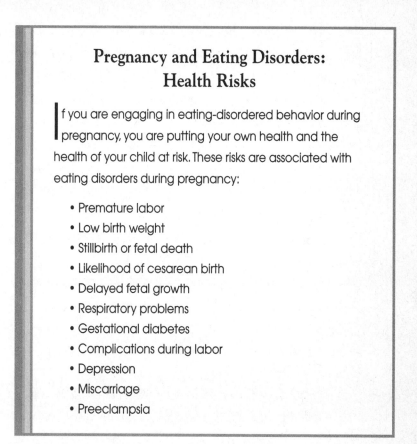

Pregnancy and Eating Disorders: Health Risks

If you are engaging in eating-disordered behavior during pregnancy, you are putting your own health and the health of your child at risk. These risks are associated with eating disorders during pregnancy:

- Premature labor
- Low birth weight
- Stillbirth or fetal death
- Likelihood of cesarean birth
- Delayed fetal growth
- Respiratory problems
- Gestational diabetes
- Complications during labor
- Depression
- Miscarriage
- Preeclampsia

Your Healthy Checklist

If you know you have food and weight issues and you want to go into motherhood prepared to deal with them, that doesn't mean you're selfish. It means you're smart, savvy, and self-aware—and we think your kids will thank you for it.

Before and During Pregnancy

✓ Discuss your plans to start a family with your doctor and/or your therapist. If you are taking antidepressants or

other medication, develop a plan that will best address
your own psychological well-being and your baby's health
through the pregnancy and beyond.

✓ Accept the basic fact that your body will go through
tremendous changes and you *will* put on pounds. If your
body-image issues and disordered eating have so far gone
untreated, now is the time to get beyond the shame and
get some help. Do not assume that these problems will
resolve themselves. Be honest with yourself and take
responsibility for your own health before you take on the
huge responsibility of motherhood.

✓ Choose an obstetrician or midwife you feel comfortable
with who is knowledgeable about eating disorders.
Disclose your eating-disorder history or any other body-
image concerns so that he or she can address any possible
risks or complications.

✓ Get your support network in place. A specialized eating-
disorders and body-image therapist can help you navigate
the emotional ups and downs of pregnancy and new
motherhood. You might also consider seeing a nutritionist
to guide you in making healthy food choices.

✓ Set boundaries with your friends, relatives, and coworkers to
minimize the talk about weight gain and other topics that could
be triggers for you. It's not easy, but start getting used to saying, "I'm not comfortable talking about that." Enlist your partner to help you steer clear of conversations and situations that
might be unhealthy for you. (see chapter 7, The WTF Files:
How to Deal with Dumb Comments and Stupid Moves).

✓ Resist the urge to shut down or close off. *Remember that there is nothing shameful about asking for help.* It's the most courageous thing you can do for yourself and your baby. Recite that one out loud. Write it on a Post-it. Send yourself a text.

After Baby Arrives

✓ Remember that your physical and emotional health are important for your baby's health. Women with histories of eating disorders have a higher risk of postpartum depression; if you are feeling depressed or anxious after the birth of your baby, do not hesitate to reach out.

✓ Just as it's important to accept that weight gain is an inevitable part of pregnancy, you also have to get comfortable with the idea that the weight you put on won't melt off the minute you give birth. If your mind is immediately racing with thoughts of getting back to the gym or dieting back into your jeans, posting your current weight on some message board under the username fattymommyblech is not as good an idea as it might seem in your sleepless-middle-of-the-night panic. Trust us on that one. You are much better off talking to a professional counselor who can help you get to a healthier place with your body issues.

✓ Look at your recovery as an ongoing process that will help you reach your full potential as an individual and as a mother. Some women find that they are able to stop their disordered-eating behavior during pregnancy while they are focusing all their attention on nurturing the baby.

However, once the baby is born or they have stopped breastfeeding, the disordered eating can return. Be ready to pick up the phone if you find yourself slipping.

Where Can I Find a Referral?

If you're looking for treatment, information, or free support groups in your area, contact the National Eating Disorders Association at 1-800-931-2237 or online at nationaleating disorders.org.

Nothing can prepare you for the exasperating challenges, hormonal roller-coaster rides, and utter exhaustion that pregnancy and new motherhood will bring into your life. But if you're getting the support and treatment you need, you'll have a better chance of weathering the storms without resorting to self-destructive habits. "There were times when I would just feel overwhelmed," recalls thirty-seven-year-old Lynda, who went to therapy throughout her pregnancy and continued to see a therapist after her son was born. "One time something happened with my son, and my husband and I had a fight. I remember being in the shower and having this strong urge to purge. I had been in recovery for my eating disorder for eighteen years and there I was in the shower thinking, 'No!' I knew consciously that I didn't want to add another problem to the problem. I chose to be in that moment and let it pass. I was developing a new identity and growing as a person and a new mom. If I had slipped back into that old behavior I would have stunted that growth. I think I was kind of arrogant before. Now I really understand that I can't take my recovery for granted. There are a lot of parallels between body image and mommy image and self-esteem and mommy esteem."

For all the minutes, hours, *days* women spend talking about food and weight, it is our silences that really hold us back. The size 2 jeans are not the key to our happiness. And deep down, we know it. So instead of discussing diet resolutions we've broken and ruminating over workout routines that aren't giving us the results we want, let's finally start getting real about what's holding us back. Let's get help if we need it and let's trade in the shame for a reality check. For our sake and the sake of our children, it's time to roll up our sleeves and support each other in finding true health and confidence.

"I have a feeling that if many women are really honest about how they see themselves, there is much room for improvement," says Sari, a forty-two-year-old mother of three daughters. The *improvement* she speaks of does not come in the form of pounds shed and calories cut—it is what happens when we open up and start those deeper conversations with ourselves and with each other.

6

Breastfeeding Is a Loaded Topic

You and your breasts go way back to puberty. Did you read *Are You There God? It's Me, Margaret* and wonder if there was even the tiniest shred of truth to those "We must increase our bust" exercises? Do you remember shopping for your first bra? Whether exciting, agonizing, or exhilarating, it was clear that things were changing when your girls first arrived on the scene.

Perhaps there have been times when you wished you could pump up your flat chest—or when you longed to subtract a few cup sizes from your ample rack. You've pushed those puppies up and you've stuffed them in. Your doctor encourages you to examine them; your partner has a grand old time groping them. You've had a lot of years to get to know your breasts. Then, during pregnancy, you might very well look down one day and wonder how someone else's gigantic ta-tas ended up on your chest. They will look different and they will feel different. You will also be reminded that mothers have been feeding their babies with these

things since the dawn of humankind. This basic biological func-
tion should not be a news flash, but you've never had to think
about if, when, and how *your* breasts would do it—until now.

Very few women are neutral on the topic of breastfeeding.
There are mothers who will give passionate speeches about how
it's the most magical bonding experience you can share with your
baby. Others will say it's painful, exhausting, and inconvenient.
Women will invite you to sign petitions to protect mothers' rights
to bare their breasts in public and others will tell you they can't
wait to stop breastfeeding. You might witness women's defenses go
up as they talk about how they never had any desire or intention
to breastfeed, and you might hear the disappointment and frustration in the voices of moms who wished they were able to, but
can't for any number of reasons.

As with most choices in the realm of pregnancy and parenting,
it can be difficult to weed through all the heightened emotions
and strong opinions when you're facing the question of whether
or not to try breastfeeding. Consult with your doctor and talk to
your partner. If you think it would be helpful to hear from your
friends or family members who have breastfed or bottlefed their
babies, by all means seek out their advice. However, at the end of
the day this is a decision you need to make with your baby's health
and your health in mind. And like your birth "plan," you can
never bank on things working out exactly as you picture them in
your ideal scenario. Just as it is not a given that every woman will
be able to conceive or deliver a baby vaginally, there are no guar-
antees about breastfeeding, either.

Breastfeeding Is Not a Breeze

Breastfeeding is far from effortless. It requires attention, coordination, and lots and lots of time. The American Academy of Pediatrics says that breastfeeding ensures the best health and development for infants. Women are often surprised when they discover what a complicated and insecurity-inducing process it can be.

"I did not feel adequately prepared at all for what breastfeeding was going to be like," says Amy, thirty-seven. "There is a lot of pressure to breastfeed and it's treated very casually in these pregnancy books. I really did not feel like I had enough information and I did not understand why breastfeeding was so hard for me. I ended up pumping 100 percent and I was going out of my mind. But things do settle down after three months and then you do kind of forget about it."

Too little information can leave women feeling unprepared for what breastfeeding entails. And too much information from the wrong sources can be just as bad, as Megan, thirty-five, learned when she started breastfeeding her baby: "I was reading some books and they said that you have to empty your breasts and it's very important that your breasts are empty. So I was trying to do everything I could to empty my breasts. I was pumping, I was hand-expressing, I was massaging my breasts and taking hot showers—basically everything the book said. And it was just so painful. It felt like my breasts were going to explode," she remembers. "Then I got sick and I had a fever. I was afraid I had mastitis, which is a disease when your milk ducts get blocked. So my partner took us to the hospital. When I told the nurse what I had been doing, she was just completely bewildered. She said, 'My God, woman! You are overstimulating yourself. Stop touching your breasts! Let your baby do her job and throw away those books you have.'"

It's easy to understand how new mothers can end up feeling unprepared or following advice that might fall short of common sense. It's a time when you're vulnerable, exhausted, and eager to provide for your child. Yet as soon as you're on your own at home after delivery, people assume that you've got everything under control. If you are trying to breastfeed and it's not going smoothly, don't blame yourself. Seek out information and support from sources you trust (see Resources at the back of this book). Call your health care provider and explain the specifics of your challenges—especially if you are worried that your baby isn't getting enough nourishment or if you are constantly in pain. Women are usually quick to pick up the phone with questions about their baby's health, but much less likely to reach out if they are the ones hurting. Don't put your own pain on the back burner, even if your baby is doing fine.

"Not Tonight, Honey. I'm Breastfeeding"

Breastfeeding can knock out your libido (see chapter 3, Let's Talk About Sex (and the) Baby). The milk-producing hormone prolactin lowers your sex drive, which is nature's way of preserving that milk supply for this baby. No nookie = no new babies to feed. You might also find that you don't want your partner coming near your breasts after that other little sucker has been all over them all day and night.

Tips for Breastfeeding Moms

1. You will have limited mobility while your baby is on the boob. Keep everything you need at arms' length by putting together a tray. Station yourself next to it when you're feeding the little one. On your tray, place the following: a giant glass or bottle of water (breastfeeding will have you believing that you've just crossed the Sahara), healthy snacks, a book or magazine to leaf through, and your cell phone with an earpiece.

2. Buy clothes in dark colors with patterns because your clothes will get stained, even if you're wearing nipple pads. Leaky breasts can be embarrassing at first, but it's something that happens to all breastfeeding mothers.

3. Remember to switch arms and switch boobs so you're not putting too much strain on one shoulder.

Busting the Breastfeeding Myths

Myth #1: Every Woman Loves Big Breasts!

"Enjoy those boobs while you've got them!" (or some variation of this) is one of the most tired and overused lines about pregnancy and breastfeeding. You'll hear it repeatedly and all those who deliver it will think they are God's gift to comedy for coming up with something so original. Yes, some women do love the natural breast enlargement that comes with pregnancy and childbearing, but many others prefer their small cups.

"I'm not a boob girl. I've always hated boobs. They got really big when I was breastfeeding. It was a little bit of a mind fuck for me to have these big jugs," remembers Zoe, thirty. "But I knew it was temporary. I knew it was for breastfeeding, which was the best thing for my child. Any time these insecurities would come up, I had to get out of my head. A crying baby who needs to eat is a good way to get out of that quickly."

Myth #2: Breastfeeding Leads to Saggy Boobs

The women we surveyed named saggy breasts as one of their top pregnancy- and motherhood-related body fears—second only to weight gain. If you are hoping to keep your breasts perky by not breastfeeding, you're out of luck. The leading causes of saggy breasts are pregnancy, time, and gravity, none of which have anything to do with breastfeeding. "It's not the breastfeeding that affects your breasts, it's the pregnancy," says Barbara Dehn, a women's health specialist. "Women who don't breastfeed also have sagging breasts. Gravity is *not* our friend." Pregnancy will change your breasts, whether you breastfeed or not. And believe it or not, so will the passage of time.

"Breastfeeding doesn't ruin your breasts! I think that aging is what causes your breasts to change," insists Mary Alice, a forty-three-year-old mother. "I'm getting older, my hormones are changing, and that affects the way my body looks."

There is no way to know ahead of time how pregnancy will change the shape of your breasts. Some women told us their breasts felt "deflated" after they stopped breastfeeding. We also heard from women whose cup size never went back to what it was before pregnancy. You could be bigger-boobed, smaller-boobed, flatter-boobed, or fuller-boobed. Wow, this is beginning to sound like a Dr. Seuss book.

Myth #3: Breastfeeding Will Make You Thin

Breastfeeding releases hormones that help the uterus contract to its original size, but it's not the key to weight loss. In fact, a study conducted by researchers Karen Wosje, Ph.D., and Heidi Kwarkof, Ph.D., RD, at the Cincinnati Children's Hospital Medical Center (published in the August 1, 2004 issue of the *American Journal of Clinical Nutrition*) showed that breastfeeding and nonbreastfeeding new mothers lost weight at similar rates and the weight decreases were not influenced by breastfeeding. La Leche League officials maintain that breastfeeding mothers lose more weight when their babies are three to six months old than formula-feeding moms, but they also state that new moms should not be focused on dieting and that crash diets and fad diets can release harmful substances into the milk supply.

We've heard many new moms singing the praises of the "breastfeeding diet." The truth is that you should eat healthy foods according to your hunger and your doctor's recommendations while you're breastfeeding. Nourish your baby and your body and let go of the idea that breastfeeding is your ticket to thinness.

Breastfeeding in Public

Nursing at home is one thing, but a lot of new moms feel intimidated to take the plunge and bare their breasts in public. Elita, 30, wrote about her "first time" on her blog (blacktating.blogspot.com) and recalled how the kindness of one stranger put her at ease: "The day came when I was in Target and the baby got hungry. . . . I had a cart full of stuff and it was raining outside and I had no alternative. I was alone and starting to get nervous, but I knew I had to do what I had to do. So I sat down in the shoe department to nurse my baby. A couple of minutes into nursing him, a German woman approached me and started talking to me. She told me how great it was that I was breastfeeding and how strange it was for her that so many people in America have hang-ups about nursing and nursing in public."

Elita says that encounter gave her the confidence to nurse "anywhere and everywhere." She stopped fearing that people would criticize her. Today she makes a conscious effort to pay that stranger's kindness forward. "When I see a mom nursing in public, I wonder if she feels the way I did that day, nervous that someone might say something to her, that she will be asked to cover up, or worse, to leave," she says. "I always at least give her a little wink or smile to show my support."

A New Perspective

Pregnancy and new motherhood give us lots of opportunities to appreciate our bodies for what they do instead of obsessing over what they look like. Breastfeeding is not about how your breasts look and, for many women, that realization can be very liberating. "As far as body image goes, I think that my body now is a lot different than before I had my son. But it is also a body that has served a purpose. I look at my belly, a little looser than before, and remind myself that it carried him while he grew. I look at my breasts, lower and less full than before, and remind myself that they nourished my tiny premature baby into a rough-and-tumble toddler," says Stephanie, twenty-six.

"Your baby doesn't care about top models or celebrities," says Anna, thirty-one. "Your baby loves you."

A Message for Girlfriends and Partners!

We know you mean well when you offer that breastfeeding new mom a heaping plate of delicious food. She's worked up an appetite taking care of that infant. But here's the thing: She can't cut up that steak while she's got a baby attached to her boob. If you want to be really nice, put together some nutritious finger foods.

Never ever dump even the smallest amount of pumped breast milk down the drain without the mother's permission. This is precious stuff! Each little bottle took a lot of time to produce and it represents several hours of freedom for the mom who pumped it.

Breast Isn't Always Best

Breastfeeding is one of the most natural human acts. That doesn't mean it comes naturally or easily to all women. There are instances when breastfeeding just isn't an option for health or lifestyle reasons, or when a mother has tried and tried and the experience is too painful or disruptive to her life and she decides to stop. Some mothers we talked to said they decided not to breastfeed because they couldn't manage it while also caring for other small children, or because they needed to go back to work right away and they could not feasibly pump breast milk throughout the day or didn't feel comfortable doing so.

"I felt a tremendous pressure to breastfeed, from the women, baby stores—everything seemed to be all about breastfeeding. It's a new world that opens itself up to you," says Peggy, thirty-two. "I didn't even know that you had to pump your breasts! I didn't even know such a thing existed. It completely made me feel like a milk cow."

For women who want to breastfeed but are unable to, the pressure can be even more overwhelming. Erica, thirty-eight, struggled to breastfeed for three weeks. "I looked at my partner one day when I was pumping, and I put down the pump and I just started to cry," she remembers. "I said, 'Baby, I hate this.' The realization finally hit that, you know what? This is not working for us. It's not working for our family. And as much as I could continue to almost self-mutilate to make it happen, it wasn't worth it." Things were made even more difficult for Erica by the fact that so many others were lining up to pass judgment on her situation.

"Everybody had an opinion and everybody wanted to tell me what I was doing wrong," she says. "I knew I was doing everything I could do to do it right and it wasn't working. So it was like, fuck you all. You don't know what I'm going through. And you know what? I've tried everything that you've brought up and it's not working. It was that stuff that was the hardest for me. It was harder than being pregnant. It was harder than the body-image stuff that goes along with pregnancy and harder than the identity stuff. It was the breastfeeding. I knew I didn't want to feel resentful when I was feeding my child."

You are the only one who can give yourself permission to stop breastfeeding if that's what you need to do. "I was in a lot of pain for a month," says Kate, thirty-two. "I would cry through the pain and my husband asked me why I didn't just stop. We got into a huge fight over this and he said that no one could tell me what to do. I decided he was right. It was my decision—an emotional one. At the one-month mark, I decided to stop. I wish more people would talk about the myth of pleasurable breastfeeding— it certainly wasn't that way for me. You feel your body is supposed to do this, and even the lactation consultants couldn't help me."

Disappointment sets in when women feel as if their bodies can't do what they're "supposed" to do. This can happen when pregnancy or childbirth doesn't go the way you expected they would, and when breastfeeding is difficult or impossible. "If the circumstances just didn't allow, then it is a loss if the mom really wanted to breastfeed," acknowledges Sherry Rumsey, a doula, birthing class instructor, and student midwife. "You're supposed to be so happy because, thank goodness, your baby is healthy. And you are happy. But you're also sad. I think too many women are expected to choke that down."

Allow yourself to go through that sense of loss if breastfeeding doesn't work out for you. And if you gave it a try, give yourself credit for the effort. "I applaud whatever a woman is able to do because every little bit counts. Just because you don't breastfeed for a year doesn't mean that the week you did breastfeed wasn't valuable. Of course it was," says Rumsey.

Rx Alert

Some medications are not safe for breastfeeding. Discuss your options with your health care provider and remember that you need to take care of your own physical and mental health to be a good parent to your child.

Magali says:

"Breastfeeding my daughter was the most intimate and rewarding feeling I've ever had. I loved it, but it was a complicated love affair. The start was very difficult, as she had to learn and I had to learn to breastfeed. The pressure to provide for her was on and the physical pain of it was unexpected. Even though I had been warned about cracked nipples and given a nipple cream, I didn't realize I had to keep breastfeeding through it. The breast pump is not easy to figure out. I pumped just about everywhere in the world—airport bathrooms, airplane bathrooms, studio bathrooms, friends' bathrooms, in the back of cabs, trailers, on the phone. Hell, I even pumped in front of girlfriends while continuing my conversations. I never had a problem pulling my shirt down or having my child pull my shirt down in public. But then again, I do come from a different culture where tits aren't exclusive to porn Web sites and Playboy bunnies.

Letting go of breastfeeding my child was very hard. It is an exclusive, tender, and time-limited experience that will never come back. The way they look up at you and into your eyes, the calm and comfort it provides them—it was worth every minute it took away from my schedule."

In Her Own Words:

I Couldn't Breastfeed

I had a breast reduction when I was nineteen. I was told at the time that I may or may not be able to breastfeed. My doctor had actually had a lot of success with his patients who went on to get pregnant and breastfeed.

Well, it didn't work. With my first pregnancy, that was devastating. The lack of support was horrible because where I live, everyone breastfeeds. I had the signs, like the tinglings and my nipples got darker, and I just assumed it would happen. And it didn't. I didn't produce any milk and I had to stop after four weeks.

The complete lack of support for how to feed a baby a bottle got to me. I didn't know anyone who was bottlefeeding. I think when you're pregnant or you've just had a baby and you've got all those hormones and your body is feeling so different, it doesn't take much. A little grain of doubt gets planted and then it takes over.

When I got pregnant with my second child, I thought I would give breastfeeding a try again. I had even more signs—my breasts got bigger during that pregnancy, which they didn't during the first. But it didn't happen. It wasn't like that black hole of depression, though. It was better. By that point, I was fed up with the lack of information out there for bottlefeeding moms. I know it sounds so basic—how hard is it? You pour the formula in the bottle, what's the problem? But there are so many different formulas out there and so many different bottles. It's not something you would instinctively know about. So as I was going through it, I wrote it all in my blog, Formula Fed and Flexible Parenting (flexibleparenting.com). It was so nice to meet other women who were in my position.

Nancy, 33

7

The WTF Files: How to Deal with Dumb Comments and Stupid Moves

You've probably heard that pregnant women and new mothers often take a turn into crazy town, where erratic mood swings and extreme nesting are ways of life. But there is another type of strange behavior that can't simply be chalked up to haywire hormones. It's what happens to everyone else when they are in the presence of an expectant or new mother. You will discover this soon, if you haven't already: Exposure to pregnancy and moms with newborns often causes otherwise rational people to say and do inexplicably inane things (and don't even get us started on the people who started out not-so-rational; they turn completely wackadoodle). These things include, but are not limited to, offering unsolicited advice, manhandling your belly, sharing their own labor and delivery horror stories, commenting on how closely you resemble any number of larger-than-life land or sea creatures, and, of course, inquiring about how much weight you've gained or lost.

You've surely witnessed one of these exchanges before. Heck, you might have even found yourself saying something to a pregnant woman or a new mom and immediately wishing for a do-over when you realize that you've just put your foot in your mouth. Many offenders have good intentions, but somehow they end up fumbling and bumbling. And then there are the truly obnoxious folks out there who will make it their business to get in other people's business—where they're not wanted and they don't belong.

If there's one thing you can count on, it's extra attention. Depending on the situation and how you're feeling at any given moment, you might enjoy some of it. It can be fun to have people gush over you, offer you seats, and dote on you as though you were the most special person in the universe. But the preggo spotlight also attracts some attention you could do without. From over-opinionated coworkers to relatives who project their own weight issues and insecurities onto you, consider this your warning that there will be moments when you'll find yourself thinking, "What the . . . ?" While you don't have much control over what other people do and say, you *do* have plenty of choices when it comes to how you handle these WTF scenarios.

Claim Your Space and Find Your Voice

Think about it. How many times have you exclaimed, "Sorry!" when someone bumps into you on a crowded street? That apologetic impulse kicks in and, for some reason, you suddenly feel compelled to excuse yourself for getting in the way, even when you're just going about your life and doing your own thing. It happens all the time, and considering how much time and energy women spend trying to make ourselves smaller and talking about how we wish various parts of our bodies were smaller, it's not all that surprising that we're so quick to take the blame. We're just not that comfortable taking up space.

Pregnancy is a whole new ball game. You will get *bigger* by the day and you will take up more space than ever. Being pregnant is in no way, shape, or form an under-the-radar kind of experience. After a certain point, people will notice you. And they will make it clear, each in their own special way, that they notice you. That level of exposure can be tough to handle—especially when it's so body-focused.

The best way to deal with all the new attention is to set some boundaries. That task doesn't come easily for most women. We are raised to be "nice" and "polite" and we will often do everything in our power to avoid disappointing others or hurting anyone's feelings, even if it means sacrificing our own well-being in the process. We learn how to put on a happy face to disguise the fact that we are annoyed or just plain pissed off.

Pregnancy is the time to let go of those people-pleasing tendencies so you can start taking care of yourself. If you don't learn how to do that now, you'll end up feeling wiped out and you'll get steamrolled by others' voices instead of listening to your own. That's not a pattern you want to keep repeating as a mom.

Speak Up for Yourself!

*"Be more verbal instead of passive. In our culture, there
is still this notion that women just don't have a voice.
Then pregnancy happens and there are all these expectations on us that we need to fulfill and it's really difficult. The more women can start to feel empowered to
have a voice, the better it will be for everyone."*

—Lesley Goth, PsyD, body-image therapist

From Weight-Gain Guessing to Tummy Touching: Five Steps to Setting Boundaries

1. **Figure out early on what you are okay with and what you're not okay with.** We'll admit that in your wildest imagi-nation, you can't begin to dream up some of the bizarro things that will come out of people's mouths during your pregnancy and after you give birth. But it does help to give some thought to the categories of comments and ques-tions that have the potential to set off insecurities or put you on the defensive. What details are you comfortable dis-cussing with whom? Just because you talk about your breastfeeding challenges with your mother doesn't mean you're obligated to share that same information with your dry cleaner if she asks.

2. **Make conversations about weight and body size off-limits.** This can be a tough one because so many women are

accustomed to talking about pregnancy weight gain and postbaby weight loss. It's healthy to ask for support when we're anxious or upset about our changing bodies, but there's a difference between sharing how we feel and trading notes on how much we've gained or lost. Unfortunately, the latter conversations are much more common. They don't really help us feel better about our bodies in the long run. Instead, they keep us trapped in the perpetual cycle of commiseration and comparison.

3. **Enlist the help of your partner, family, and friends.** This one requires you to go beyond *thinking* about your boundaries—you have to *specify them out loud.* Don't worry, you're not required to make some big, dramatic announcement. When your girlfriend is gushing about how excited she is for you, it's a good time to add, "Hey, it would be great if you could run interference if you see me getting quizzed about my weight. I've decided I just don't want to get into it." Entrusting your loved ones to be on the lookout is also a good way to encourage them to be on their best behavior, too.

4. **Pick your battles.** Let's face it. If your batty great aunt Judith hasn't changed her attitude in ninety years, she's probably not going to start exercising restraint and sensitivity any time soon. There are some times when a confrontation will probably be more of a headache than it's worth. But if you've made your boundaries clear to your inner circle, you'll find those encounters easier to deal with than if you were flying

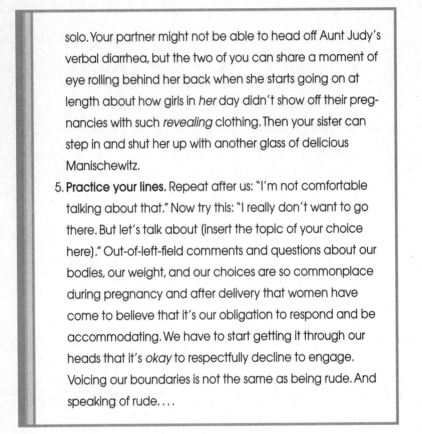

solo. Your partner might not be able to head off Aunt Judy's verbal diarrhea, but the two of you can share a moment of eye rolling behind her back when she starts going on at length about how girls in *her* day didn't show off their pregnancies with such *revealing* clothing. Then your sister can step in and shut her up with another glass of delicious Manischewitz.

5. **Practice your lines.** Repeat after us: "I'm not comfortable talking about that." Now try this: "I really don't want to go there. But let's talk about (insert the topic of your choice here)." Out-of-left-field comments and questions about our bodies, our weight, and our choices are so commonplace during pregnancy and after delivery that women have come to believe that it's our obligation to respond and be accommodating. We have to start getting it through our heads that it's *okay* to respectfully decline to engage. Voicing our boundaries is not the same as being rude. And speaking of rude....

The Top Offenders

1. The Foot-in-Mouth All-Stars

These are the people who will loudly exclaim, "Are there *twins* in there?" as if to announce that you are way too enormous to be pregnant with just one child. They have also been known to ask new moms pushing strollers when they are due. Duh! We recommend a Stephen Colbert–style incisive stare/arched eyebrow combo for these All-Stars. Make them shake in their boots a little.

2. The Tummy Touchers

Talk about touchy-feely. It's a shame they don't make electrified fences for pregnant bellies. When you see some random person's paws coming at you, you might not be able to zap them, but you are well within your rights to take a giant step back. If you're in a situation where you don't mind being touched but you *do* mind people's assumptions that they can put their hands on you whenever they please, say so before the grabfest begins: "I don't mind if you want to feel the baby kick, but just ask me first."

3. The Horror Show Oversharers

"OMG. I was in labor for three days and everything that could possibly go wrong went wrong. The pain! The gore! Let me start at the beginning. . . ."

If you are visibly pregnant, you might hear one or several of these—not because you asked one of your closest friends or family members to share her birth story with you, but because the lady in the grocery store used her keen observation skills to determine your status and felt compelled to tell you all about her nightmare of a labor in the express lane.

"You can give the nod or mm-hmm," recommends Sherry Rumsey, a doula, student midwife, and birthing class instructor. "If you want, you can ask that person, 'Is there anything you would have done differently?' That way you can see if you can actually get something useful out of what she's telling you." And don't forget that every encounter with an Oversharer should be followed by your own private pep talk, in which you remind yourself that your labor and delivery will be just that—yours.

4. The Know-It-Alls

Need to know everything there is to know about how your next-door neighbor cured her yeast infections with a remedy she concocted using herbs from her very own garden? We didn't think so. But she will tell you anyway, and she'll probably choose exactly the moment when you're feeling most exhausted and overwhelmed to share her seemingly endless expertise. Keep in mind that Know-It-Alls also have all the *time* in the world to convince you that their way is the right way. For the quickest escape, you can respectfully acknowledge their experience—"It's great that you had such positive results with that"—without actually committing to trying anything they recommend.

5. The Judges

Whereas the Know-It-Alls will tell you all about what you should be doing, the Judges are on a mission to point out what you *shouldn't* be doing—and they have the ability to make even the most pregnant of pregnant women feel incredibly small. Pregnancy and new motherhood are times when women already feel exposed and prone to self-doubt. To make matters worse, these Judges will gleefully line up to question everything from your food and beverage choices ("Should you be eating that sushi?" "I hope that's decaf!") to the items on your baby registry ("Are you sure you want that brand of baby monitor?").

Before your middle finger starts to twitch, it's important to get clear on something for yourself. Are you making informed choices about your health and your baby's health? If so, you do not have to justify those choices to anyone else. How you articulate that is up to you—and it will probably vary depending on who the Judge is—but above all else, stand firm in the knowledge that you're doing your best and there is no way in the world you can please everyone. Once you stop trying, you'll discover that it's a lot easier to brush off the people who are out to put you down.

In Her Own Words:

The WTF Hall of Fame

When I was pregnant, I had some guy in the elevator tell me, "Oh, I see you're dropping." Why, why, why would you say that? Homeless guys on the street yelled, "It's a boy!" People called me Juno.

I went to suspend my membership at the pool because I was giving birth soon and the woman at the front desk said, "What?" And she came from behind the counter to make sure I was pregnant. "I would never think that you're pregnant! Usually you can tell in someone's face that they are pregnant." But it's not like she even knows me. It was all really strange.

A lot of people give you compliments or congratulations or share their stories, which can be nice. But there is definitely a lot of focus on the fact that you're pregnant, your shape, what you're going to go through.

I don't see my father much and when he came for a visit, he said, "Where are your breasts?" This was about a month after the baby was born. I guess he was expecting an even bigger change. People just comment away—there is no hiding.

Anna, 35

Magali says:

"When I was about six months pregnant, I was flying home after a job. I noticed this man eyeing me the entire flight. As soon as we landed, he came right over to me and started telling me that he was a doctor and my thyroid looked rather big. Had I been to have it checked? It could be really dangerous for the growing fetus! He went on and on about what a big neck I had and how worried he was and how worried I should be. It seemed like that airplane door took a millennium to open. I knew logically that he was completely nuts. I had my own doctor and this guy should have been minding his own business. But I was frozen in that moment. I just waited patiently for him to finish talking and I politely exited the plane, trying hard not to reveal how deeply unsettled I was. Outside, before my car arrived, a woman came to sit next to me. She said she had been on the flight and overheard the mad doctor's monologue. She tried to offer some reassurance that he had been way out of line. I thanked her, got in my car, and headed home. But I broke down and cried on the way. I cried because I was overwhelmed. I cried because I was tired and hungry. And I cried because I was utterly humiliated. It was as though I had gone from being me—a person with feelings—to being this exposed Pregnant Body. I realized how unprepared I was to protect myself from attention I didn't want. One insensitive stranger had the power to shake my confidence completely. That woke me up and pissed me off."

How to Deal: Comments from Strangers

If we asked you to name the loudmouthed, undermining, and clueless people in your life, you could probably put together a list within a few minutes. Now we can tell you to review your list and prepare accordingly, because it's very likely that those are the folks who will fit into at least one of the Top Offender categories.

With strangers, we don't have the luxury of prep time. The bad news is that there's no telling when one of them will come out of the woodwork. The good news is that strangers don't know us. We don't owe them anything and we'll probably never see them again. So as long as you're not pulling any Mexican wrestler moves on the woman at the bookstore who insists she can tell you're having a boy because "You're carrying so small!" you'll face no consequences should you choose to put her in her place.

Jen, thirty-two, says there were a few times during her pregnancy when she just couldn't keep her exasperation to herself. "I would get on the subway and people would size me up. They would look me up and down as though they were trying to figure out if I was fat or pregnant. A couple of times I would be tired enough or mad enough to actually say, 'I'm fat *and* pregnant. You're right on both accounts. Now can you move so I can have a seat?'"

Really?

"Once I was on the beach and I was six months pregnant in a bikini. I mean seriously, I felt like I looked pregnant. We met some people and we were chatting with them. I have a tattoo on my stomach and this guy said to me, 'What would you do if you got pregnant with that tattoo? What would happen to it?' I said, 'I am pregnant! This is what I would do!' and he said, 'Oh, I thought you just had a big

beer gut.' Well, that sucked. We all kind of laughed but then I thought,
mental note to self: Tell everyone you're pregnant."   —Amy, 37

"I needed to use the restroom during a dinner at a restaurant and
politely asked the woman at the next table to move her chair so I
could get by. She glared at me and replied, 'Why don't you lose some
weight?' I was five months pregnant at the time and just starting to
really show. I was devastated."   —Jessica, 33

Not all comments from strangers are so dim-witted or mean-
spirited. And depending on how you're feeling, a comment that
could set you off one day might amuse you or even comfort you
the next.

"I remember going to the gym two or three months after having the baby and everyone was saying to me, 'Oh my God, it's the
best to have a baby! Isn't it the best?' I thought, *Really? I don't
think it's the best. This is so hard,*" says Marian, thirty-six. "And
then some guy walked over—he was a total bachelor—and he
said, 'Children are overrated.'" Rather than getting offended,
Marian says his blunt statement actually filled her with a sense of
relief that someone else had stepped in to burst that "perfect,
happy mommy" bubble.

The Bottom Line: When dealing with strangers, remember
that you have no relationship with them to nurture or protect. If
you don't want to answer someone's prying questions, you can say
so with relatively low risk of ever coming into contact with that
person again. If someone hurts your feelings or says something
rude, you can give that person a piece of your mind and then walk

away. In Jessica's case, we would have recommended calling the waiter over to notify him of the horrendous odor wafting over from the next table—because people who feel the need to insult others really do stink.

How to Deal: Comments from Coworkers

If you work in an office, you probably see your coworkers more than you see your own family. Perhaps you're lucky enough to have some colleagues you actually enjoy spending time with. However, the fact that every workplace is essentially a random mix of quirks and personalities means that you can count on receiving some crazy comments as soon as your pregnancy becomes a hot topic at the water cooler.

You'll have to learn how to handle these comments wearing your professional hat. So while you might be looking at your boss, thinking, *WTF?* when she suggests that the janitor's closet at the end of the hall might be the perfect private space for you to pump breast milk during the workday, you would be wise not to voice those three words out loud. Take the issue up with human resources instead. Unless the human resources manager is an offender herself, which is not unheard of.

Rachel, twenty-nine, thirteen weeks pregnant, was accosted by her company's HR manager, who walked right up to her in the office, rubbed her belly, and asked her how far along she was. "She told me how she had kept her pregnancy hidden until past fifteen weeks—to the point when her boss asked a coworker of hers whether she was pregnant, as she seemed to have gained some weight. There were so many things inappropriate about this I don't even know where to start," Rachel says. "The best part certainly was that it was our HR manager! We do not have the sort of close or friendly relationship that would make it anything but very odd for her to walk up and rub my tummy."

And that wasn't the only office offender Rachel encountered. "One of the funniest ones happened in a one-on-one meeting with a colleague," she remembers. "She suddenly said—without any context—that my face was changing. She was clearly excited and awaiting my response, so I said I hadn't noticed. She pressed on that. Yes, it was becoming fuller and hadn't my husband said anything? The whole exchange went on just a bit longer, and it gave some of my friends and me fodder for lots of giggles. How can I possibly fit my giant face through the door these days?"

Really?!?

"At my office baby shower, coworkers were asking questions like, 'How are you feeling?' and 'How's the house?' and one coworker, who has children, asked me how much weight I had gained! I tried to dodge it by saying that I had gained in the zone of what I should weigh and she said, 'No, how much?' I felt called on it, on the spot, in public. And I answered—22 pounds. She said, 'Good for you!' like it was an accomplishment. That was a little WTF."

—Paula, 38

"I have one coworker who has something to say about everyone and everything—a real know-it-all. I see her every day and every day she would have something to say. She'd say things like, 'Oh yeah, you're definitely having a boy, you got round all over' or 'This baby is definitely a boy, you got so big all over' or 'It's definitely a boy because you're carrying just the way I did when I was carrying my son. My boobs got big, my butt got big, my belly was big, I was just big all over!' At this point I wanted to be really obnoxious and say to her that I guess she's still carrying all that extra weight since giving birth to her son—who is forty—but I thought better of it. That would have been pretty funny, though. And for the record, we're having a girl. So I guess Miss Know-It-All doesn't know everything!"

—Kerri, 37

The Bottom Line: Keep your cool. Remember that you can respectfully and professionally decline to discuss your pregnancy or parenting choices with coworkers. If a situation is truly making you feel unsafe or uncomfortable, raise the issue with someone who is in a position to help you (in Rachel's case, we recommend going straight to the top of the food chain; clearly her HR department is in desperate need of sensitivity training). And don't forget to blow off some steam by laughing about these workplace doozies when you can. Launching into an angry tirade at the office won't be good for your career, but feel free to poke fun at your coworkers' WTF comments with your friends and family.

How to Deal: Comments from Your Family, Your Friends, and Your Partner

When someone on the street says you look like you're about to burst, it's annoying enough. When your own mother says you look like you're "pregnant in your ass," that sting radiates much deeper. Comments and criticisms from the people we are closest to are the ones that can hurt us the most. It's tough to brush off these exchanges because they remind us that whatever insecurities we have, they were not created in a vacuum. And if the comments are related to our size or our weight, they reinforce the cycle of body issues in our past and our present. But that cycle can stop with us.

If you are sensitive about your weight and your body image, establish ground rules with your family, your friends, and your partner early in your pregnancy and make it clear that you can't tolerate any critiques or "jokes" about your body during pregnancy and after delivery. It's also a good idea to identify the likely offenders. If they are aware of your boundaries and can't manage to respect them, you owe it yourself and your baby to minimize your exposure to that bad energy. "My mother has been critical of my weight since I was a teenager. I try to just ignore it. Happily, she lives a thousand miles away!" says Molly, thirty-seven, in her ninth week of pregnancy.

Even without a large buffer zone, you can still create distance if you need it. Ask for help from those supportive people in your life who do have your back. "My mother's comments have been so relentless that nearly all of my family, including my partner, have felt the need to remonstrate with her about it. My friends, hearing some of the comments, have expressed the wish to do the same," says Heather, thirty-two, in her twenty-fifth week of pregnancy. "It also makes me extremely likely to eat whole packets of cookies immediately after seeing her. These comments continued into pregnancy, with a lecture about not putting on weight by eating for two. And then I was sick for weeks and weeks and lost a lot of weight and never got my appetite back. She seems content. Everyone else worried."

Let's get real here. If dealing with someone in your family is triggering disordered eating, anxiety, or any other unhealthy behaviors, it's time to put on the brakes and pay attention to that giant red flag in front of you. You need to take care of yourself. If there are people in your life who can't support you in that—in the way *you're* asking them to support you, not in the way *they* think is best—you have to take a giant step back until they can deal with their issues. Trust us, these are *their* issues. They don't have to continue to be your issues and those issues certainly don't have to be passed on to your children.

Really?!?

"I feel like my parents are being judgmental. They even think my dog and cat are fat, which they are not."   —Melissa, 33

"My mother-in-law called me fat, which made me feel awful about myself."   —Amanda, 33, at 38 weeks pregnant

"My dad would often say, 'Ah, you've gained some weight,' or, when looking at old pictures, he would say, 'You were kind of fat then.' When I haven't lost a lot of weight, he won't say anything about how I look. It's only when I do lose weight that he'll say I look good."

—Liz, 39, at 14 weeks pregnant

"My mom frames her comments in the form of 'helpful' eating and dieting tips, in addition to paying special attention to what I'm eating. She would never say something overt about my weight, but instead focuses on what she feels is the best way to eat to lose weight. She's also keenly interested in what my nutritionist says and lets me know whether or not she agrees with her. I also recall a couple of instances where my mom has mentioned how important it is to 'get proactive' about losing baby weight; otherwise it sticks around for a while.

"My dad would never say anything to me overtly, but he is obsessed with my younger sister's weight. She is overweight and he can't stop talking about how it's affecting her ability to get a good job, get pregnant, etc. When I started to get heavy as well, in between my pregnancies, I found it interesting that he didn't stop this kind of talk, but rather escalated it around me. I can't bring myself to say to them, 'Don't worry, I'm going to get to a healthy weight again after the baby' because it's none of their business and they should have faith in my ability to take care of myself. But, of course, the fact that we don't outwardly talk about this stuff makes for a lot of resentment."

—Ann, 40

Family Drama

There are certain topics related to pregnancy, birth, and parenting that can end up in heated family debate. If you already know what those issues will be, start thinking about how you'll handle them. Breastfeeding, circumcision, and birth plans are three of the biggies.

"I tell people that you don't have to tell family members or friends what your plans are if you think they're not going to be supportive of your choice," says Sherry Rumsey, a doula, student midwife, and birthing class instructor. "I had a couple who planned a home birth and they didn't tell any of their family until after the baby was born. They called their parents and said, 'We had the baby at home!' They knew that their family would not be supportive of that choice and they just didn't want to go down that road."

If you do want to fill in your family and friends ahead of time, but want to exercise control over the situation, Rumsey recommends putting your decision in writing. "If you know there's going to be a big issue, type up a letter about why you are choosing what you are choosing. You can invite people to present you with research that supports their opinion, but you need to make it clear that this is your decision," she says.

With Friends Like These

Friends—even the ones who have been with us through thick and . . . make that good and bad—have been known to say things that put you down and put you on guard. "I know my friends don't mean to say I am fat when they joke that it looks like I am either further along than they think or I have more than one baby. But it still hurts," says Nicki, nineteen.

Don't swallow that last sentence or push it down. Whatever our friends' intentions, it's up to us to make it clear that their words *do* hurt. That's how they'll learn what they should and shouldn't say to you (and any other pregnant women, for goodness sake!) in the future.

You will find that pregnancy and new motherhood are times that can bring out the best in some of your friends and the worst in others. Bonds will be strengthened and bonds will be broken.

"I wish my college friends, who were really my sisterhood, would have told me that my baby shower was really a going-away party," says Jen, thirty-two. "It would have been better to have been prepared than to be shocked by that. That really was the end of the friendship. That was the last time I saw them and felt like we were remotely the same friends. It was painfully clear that they didn't want to hear about my new life. Not only did they not want to know about it, but they didn't want to give me an opportunity to talk about something else. It was like this assumption that I would have nothing else to talk about."

Women who are the first among their friends to become moms speak of feeling left out or misunderstood. Women who are the last among their friends to have children speak of feeling left behind or ignored. And women who have friends with children the same age as their children speak of feeling in competition and insecure. It's complicated, to say the least. But when it comes down to it, we need the ebb and flow of these friendships in our lives. We come to understand the unique support each person can give us, and what we can give in return. The dynamic of each friendship sustains us in a different way. We can choose whom we call to ask which question. We can choose what friend we need to avoid when we're feeling sensitive, but who we can always turn to when we need a dose of tell-it-like-it-is. We can choose—and because we know our friends, we can choose wisely.

Teasing That Hurts

Offhanded comments or "lighthearted" jabs about our changing bodies aren't all that funny when we're feeling insecure. The biggest offenders in this department? Partners.

"Both my six-year-old and my husband have made comments about how big they think I look, which is so not helpful."

—Jane, 32, at 34 weeks pregnant

"My partner commented on me being massive and worrying that it's twins!"   —Katy, 32, at 11 weeks pregnant

"My husband keeps talking enthusiastically about my new 'fat' body, which makes me twitch a bit."   —Heather, 32, at 25 weeks pregnant

Some partners are completely floored by the body changes of pregnancy. "The biggest surprise for me was learning how much I didn't know. I didn't know anything about how a woman's body changes during pregnancy," recalls Scott, 49. "I just had no

cognizance about the whole process and how detailed it all is."
This level of shock and awe has been known to cause some foot-
in-mouth behavior. If your partner makes a comment that doesn't
feel so supportive, offer the benefit of the doubt for a first offense,
speak up, and ask for the kind of support you do need.

The Bottom Line: In a perfect world, your friends, your family,
and your partner would know better than to criticize your weight
or tease you about the size of your body—in general and *especially*
during pregnancy and after delivery when you might be extra sensitive about these issues. But sometimes you really have to spell it
out for them. If people you care about slip up and cross the line,
all you should need to say is, "That hurt my feelings." And if they
still don't get it? Well, then it's time to explain why you need to
surround yourself with people who do.

How to Deal: Comments from Doctors

Your relationship with your health care providers should be
built on trust. When you choose obstetricians, midwives, and
other health care providers, you want to know that they are looking out for your best interests. You want to feel that they're on
your side. Sadly, we heard from many women who ended up in the
examination room—and sometimes even the delivery room—
feeling shamed and unsupported by their own doctors.

Really?!?

"My entire life I've felt fat . . . and unfortunately the men in my life, and my own mother, have continued to convince me that my own body is not good enough. My obstetrician was very direct with me. She hardly let me gain any weight. So, luckily, I threw up every day. I went through labor for 72 hours . . . and I had to have an emergency C-section. The C-section came with a lot of 'just in case' warnings that dealt with the fact that I was 'obese.' I swear they used that word two hundred times while telling me why I was at risk during the C-section."

—Amy, 32

"I developed a thyroid condition that was undetected during my pregnancy. I was an athlete and in the best shape of my life before conceiving. I was muscular and had a very low fat content. The male OB did not seem to believe me when I brought in my eating plan and showed him. His remark was that I must have forgotten the five chocolate bars I had eaten. I was so shocked I never discussed my weight concerns after that point."

—Yvette, 40

"I'm using a midwife, which has been great. They don't make me get on a scale so I have no idea how much weight I've gained. I eat healthy, exercise regularly—what my body does after that I have no control over and I'm grateful the midwife has an enlightened view. The two times I've been to an OB/GYN practice I was given infor-mation on pregnant women and BMI (Body Mass Index) being too high. I thought, Wow, you're telling a pregnant woman that she is too fat! How do you tell a pregnant woman to go on a diet? *Most women feel so fat and awkward anyway. To add that medical burden into the mix just floors me!"*

—Becky, 32

If your health care provider is looking at the number on the scale more than he or she is looking into your eyes and listening to what you have to say, we strongly urge you to find another doctor (see chapter 5, Adding Up, Weighing In, and Counting Down). Women with weight worries, poor body image, or histories of disordered eating deserve doctors who will treat those issues with sensitivity and treat you with respect—whether you're overweight, underweight, or normal weight.

From Queen for a Day to Get Out of the Way!

During your pregnancy, people will regularly fall all over themselves to offer you assistance, ask you how you're doing, and express their genuine interest in everything from how you're decorating the nursery to what baby names you're considering. People will gush over you, give up their seats for you, and offer to help carry your bags. Then, if all goes well, you will give birth and come home with your newborn. Roughly a few weeks later, you will venture out into the world again—this time with a stroller or a baby carrier—only to discover how drastically things have changed.

"When you're pregnant, everyone opens doors for you, picks up things for you, and brings you food. I loved it. It makes you feel like a princess!" remembers Hermione, forty-four. "But when you've got a child in a stroller, they run to get in front of you and elbow you out of the way, trying to get through to the door before you've gotten in. I know because I've been the other person kicking through the door like 'Shit, there's a woman with a stroller.'"

Yes, it's true. You are now "that woman" with the screaming infant. The one who is trying to get out of the parking lot, just like everybody else, but who must first fold the stroller, fasten the newborn into the car seat, retrieve the wallet and latte from the top of the car (a key step in the process, yet one that is often skipped), and rifle for the keys while enduring the honking horns and harsh stares of everyone in the immediate vicinity. Is it obvious that one of us has personal experience? Don't despair. Every new mother goes through this. It takes a while to get your bearings and to learn to give others the heads-up that you'll be at least ten minutes loading and unloading. You will gain new insight into how impatient and self-important some people can be. On the plus side, these experiences will definitely help you build thicker skin.

A Message for Girlfriends!

Ask your friend if she wants company on her first few outings with the baby. Some moms like to test the waters to see what they can handle on their own, but others will eagerly accept an extra pair of helping hands!

Smart Moves: New Mom Meal Delivery

If you've ever been struck by how dramatically the attention shifts from the pregnant woman to the new baby, you're not alone. Hey, we get it. Babies are pretty irresistible. In all the "oohing and ahhing," we've seen mothers go through major attention withdrawal. It must be a rude awakening when those months of special treatment come to a screeching (and shrieking) halt. Here's an idea we tried recently, which gives some love and tasty goodness back to the moms.

1. Pass around a sign-up sheet at the baby shower and ask for volunteers who can prepare and deliver a nutritious meal to the parents during their first week with their newborn. Each volunteer should provide a phone number and e-mail address so you can follow up.

2. Find out what foods are the parents' favorites and what foods they're allergic to or just find generally disgusting. You don't want them to end up with a tray full of tuna casserole if it's going to turn their stomachs.

3. Once you know when the new family will be home from the hospital, organize a drop-off schedule with your volunteers. Make sure all those who signed up are clear that they should deliver the food and run. This isn't the time to visit unless you are specifically invited in—and if you are, don't linger too long.

Magali says:

"Even when it feels like you've been downgraded to chopped liver status once the baby arrives, if you listen very closely, you will detect the sweet sounds of people offering to help. Sometimes that lifetime use of the 'No, I'm fine' autoreply can drown out the message we all desperately need to hear as new moms. People still care! They want to know if there's anything we need! So reset your autoreply to 'Yes, please.'"

"Yes, please!"

Question: Do you need anything?

Answer: Yes, please! In my fridge I have. . . . But I could use some. . . .

Question: Can I come by to see the baby?

Answer: Yes, please! How about tomorrow? It's hard to predict when he/she and I will be awake, but pick up some [favorite beverage] and [snack of choice] and we'll hang out for as long as I can manage. You're welcome to make calls, pay your bills, or surf the worldwide interwebs while I drift in and out of consciousness/coherence.

Question: Can I bring you anything?

Answer: Yes, please!

Pick from the following:

- A trashy novel
- The current issue of your favorite magazine (Ix-nay on the tabloids with "Miracle Mommy Makeover" stories!)
- Fresh flowers for the house
- A movie
- Takeout from your favorite restaurant
- A beauty treat

The Perfect Comeback

When you are on the receiving end of a WTF comment or a stupid move, you will no doubt be able to dream up the most jaw-dropping zinger of a comeback that fits the situation perfectly.

Sadly, that will usually happen several hours later, after the encounter is long over and the offender long gone. Unless you are Don Rickles (in which case, we would really have to question how you ended up pregnant and why you are reading this book), expect to be thrown off guard and thrown for a loop on more than one occasion. And that's okay. You don't need the wittiest responses—you just need responses that get your point across and keep you from getting into conversations that are unhealthy for you.

A Response for Every WTF

Pick from this handy list or tailor your own responses, depending on which offender you're facing down.

- "Uh-oh, time to pee again! Where's the closest bathroom?"
- "I can't tell you how much weight I've gained/lost, but I can tell you I'm fine and the baby is fine, too."
- "I'm not comfortable talking about that."
- "I don't want to go there."
- "That hurt my feelings."
- "There are lots of different expert opinions on this issue. We'll have to agree to disagree."
- "Oh, was that a joke? Sorry, I didn't get it."
- "I'm smiling with my eyes right now. Can you tell? Do you see the smile? How about now?" (Hopefully by this point the offender is nervously backing up or breaking into a run—away from you.)
- "Hmmm. Fascinating. Bye-bye."
- Or you can test out a classic line that always seemed to work so well on *Full House*: "How rude!"

8

Feeling Beautiful for Two: Why Healthy Body Image Will Make You a Better Mother

You'll hear a lot about balance when you start talking to moms. Schedules, relationships, and career goals must be balanced with the new responsibilities of parenthood. People will tell you that there is no effortless route to having it all. In fact, many would argue that "having it all" belongs in the same category as "riding a magic unicorn to the end of the rainbow." But no matter what you believe about the road to balance, your life *will* be different when you become a parent—and you will have to work at making it work.

Women are beginning to understand that living a life of rigid extremes just doesn't jibe with being a mom. And we're getting better at owning up to the challenges of juggling our many roles.

Except, that is, when we start talking about our looks. Unfortunately, while we learn about the importance of "compromises," "priorities," and "flexibility"—all of which serve to remind women that there is a give-and-take to this mothering thing—we're simultaneously seeing a proliferation of new catchphrases like *prebaby body*, *mommy makeover*, and *postbaby weight loss*. Instead of figuring out how to redefine beauty to fit our new lives and how to accept (and maybe even embrace) the changes in our bodies, mothers and mothers-to-be are more and more frequently finding themselves obsessing over one question: "How will I get my body back?"

Finding Your Beauty-Baby Balance

Think about the term *work-life balance*. For working moms, it's practically a mantra because the concept is grounded in the idea that (gasp!) we have to make some adjustments and sometimes even some sacrifices to find balance. So we develop new strategies to live our lives—as mothers, as partners, and as individuals. We don't always get it exactly right, but we do try our best. "Being a mom is the ultimate challenge in learning how to balance your life," says Gina, forty-two. "Falling in love with your child can change how you see the world and yourself."

What if we aimed to achieve that kind of balance and perspective with our bodies? Just because you can't work out six days a week like Gwyneth Paltrow doesn't mean you are doomed to become a mom who lets herself go. And if your less-than-taut stomach is bothering you today, that doesn't mean you need to call up a plastic surgeon tomorrow. Yet somehow, in our out-of-balance world, these extremes have become acceptable solutions and ideals we constantly measure ourselves against.

"We want women to be unbelievably skinny, unbelievably beautiful, be able to work eighty hours a week, and also be home for a hundred hours a week, to wear stiletto heels and also be on the soccer field. It's not possible. The only ones who can manage to portray that it is possible are people with millions of dollars. They don't have it all, but we're expected to believe they do," says Jen, thirty-two.

The Beauty-Baby Balance Principles

Take Time for Yourself
"Let it be. Don't get so lost in being a mom that you lose you. Take time for yourself when you can. It is the healthiest thing you can do for you and your family."
—Michele, 33

Take Care of Yourself
"Happy moms have happy babies. You can't neglect yourself. By taking care of yourself, both physically and mentally, you are directly taking better care of your child."
—Tanya, 34

Tune Out the Media Static and Tune into Yourself
"Do not buy into the myth that you have to get your body back quickly like the stars in the media do. You are more than just a pretty face. You have things to contribute. Pregnancy is a time to tap into all the female wisdom you have inside. It is a time to reflect on what you think and feel is important."
—Yvette, 40

The Legacy of Body Hatred:
Breaking the Cycle

You want your children to grow up feeling strong in who they are. As a parent, you are a provider, a teacher, and a protector; if you have struggled with body hatred, you will probably give a lot of thought to how you will protect your children from going through those same struggles.

"I have two girls and I definitely don't ever want to feel that way again because I don't want them to feel that energy or feel like they can't eat anything because it will make them fat," worries Cassandra, a thirty-three-year-old mother with a history of bulimia. "I do not want to inflict any of that old life of mine onto them because that was not a happy time. I would never want them to go through that."

When you start thinking about the kind of messages about food, weight, and body image you want to give to your children, the next logical step is to reflect on the messages you received growing up. For many women, what they heard and observed was far from healthy.

"Throughout late elementary and middle school, I had an extremely restrictive diet (existed on sugar-free Jell-O and diet sodas), and I frequently binged and purged," recalls Emily, twenty-four. "I had a mother who was always on a diet and parents who were 'concerned about my health,' which of course meant my 'weight.' I was wearing a size 12. I always associated getting thinner with being happy, getting a boyfriend, having more friends, being more glamorous, and I was very insecure about my size. In college I learned more about health at any size. I realized that I lived a healthy, active lifestyle, and that the body I have *is* healthy, despite what other people think."

Janet, thirty-five and eighteen weeks pregnant with her first child, describes herself as having a history of bulimia in high school and "just typical adult female body issues—always about twenty pounds overweight, but I see myself as about eighty pounds overweight." Her parents didn't exactly boost her self-esteem as a child. "My mom and dad called me fat names during my adolescence. My dad offered to pay me to lose weight—he offered thousands of dollars, clothes, and cars. He gave a very conditional message about love."

The wounds from that kind of shaming and verbal abuse run deep, and the emotional roller coaster of pregnancy and new motherhood can reopen them. If you want to protect your child, the first thing you need to do is protect yourself. Set boundaries (see chapter 7, "The WTF Files") with the people in your life who make you feel insecure and if you need to, minimize the time you spend with them. You and your children don't have to live with the burden of someone else's issues, but it's up to you to get help for yourself so you can start healing those wounds.

As mothers and mothers-to-be, we can't stop the legacy of body hatred unless we start a new legacy of body confidence. There will be times when we fall short and bad body-image days when we will judge ourselves harshly. We will have moments when we're sure we've messed up our kids forever, too. Our parents didn't get it exactly right and neither will we. But we have to keep trying our best to accept and appreciate our bodies so we can teach our children to accept and appreciate theirs.

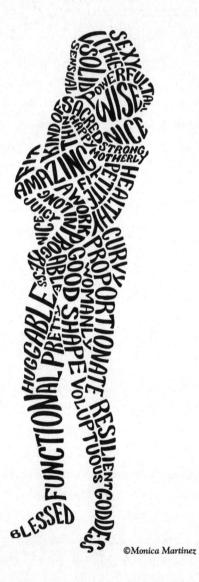

©Monica Martinez

The way we see ourselves has a direct impact on our children. We asked mothers to tell us what words they use to describe their bodies. This is what they shared.

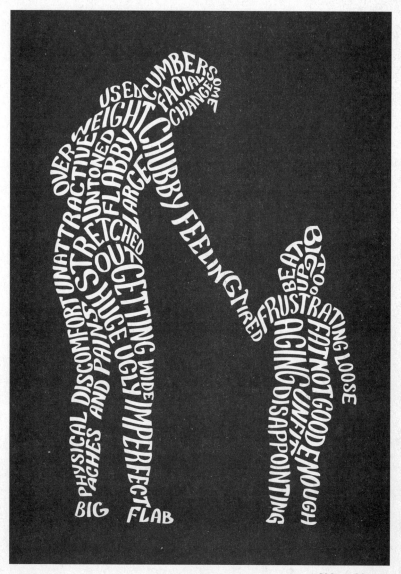

©Monica Martinez

Teens at Risk

In a five-year study of more than 2,500 teenagers, researchers at the University of Minnesota found that 44 percent of girls and 29 percent of boys were overweight, habitual binge eaters, or had taken unhealthy measures to lose weight—such as abusing laxatives, using diet pills, or vomiting. In particular, being teased by a family member appeared to raise the risk of all three problems in girls. Among the other risk factors were a preoccupation with weight, having a mother who dieted, and frequently reading magazine articles on weight loss.

Eating Disorders: Genetic Roots

There is research that shows that eating disorders have genetic and biological roots. Some women with a history of eating disorders choose not to have biological children because they are concerned about passing their illness on to their child, or they are worried that the body changes of pregnancy would be too stressful for them. This is a personal and incredibly difficult decision—and we respect any woman for being in tune to what is right for her. There are many other eating-disorder sufferers who go on to have happy and healthy babies (Magali is one of them). What's most important is to find compassionate health care providers and get extra support (see chapter 5, Adding Up, Weighing In, and Counting Down).

It's More Than Just "Faking It": Teaching Healthy Habits and Attitudes to Our Children

Body hatred doesn't just come out in the things women *say*. It is evident in the way we carry ourselves, the food we eat, the sidelong glances at reflective surfaces, and the sighs of exasperation or resignation. It is also revealed in the clothes we wear, try on, and return; the desserts we refuse; and the repeated trips to the scale. If you are struggling to accept your body, you are *living* that struggle—in your words, your actions, and your attitude. Even if you think you are the queen of deception and you have everyone fooled, body hatred has many tells.

We would love to live in a world where all women get healthy by working to get their body-image issues in check before they become moms, instead of trying to diet down to an "ideal weight" before pregnancy. It would be encouraging to see pregnant women preparing for their new lives, not stressing over pregnancy weight gain. And how amazing would it be if every new mother could take the time to heal and find her footing instead of immediately worrying about "getting her body back"? Unfortunately, we don't live in that world—at least not yet. There are plenty of pregnant women and new mothers who are just beginning to understand why it is important to let go of body hatred if they want to help their children resist the very real pressures that exist in this world.

No matter where we are in the process, it's never too late to pay attention to how we are affected by body insecurities. Yes, we do need to be mindful about what we say about our bodies in front of children—but if we're serious about getting healthy, we need to be mindful about how we treat our bodies in *every* facet of our lives. We can't just "fake" body confidence when our children are around and continue to dwell on our insecurities everywhere else.

"I always remember my mom being encouraging and supportive. Yet, at the same time, I don't think she was able to live it as much as she was able to talk it, so there is definitely a disconnect when you're getting that mixed message," says Lisa, thirty-two.

It's important for your children to understand that you put a higher value on good health than you do on weight or physical appearance. When you stop yourself from making a comment about your sagging stomach in front of your child, you're not "pretending" that insecurity doesn't exist; you're acknowledging to yourself that it's not something you want your child to absorb. When you eat the same dinner as your children instead of the salad they might be used to seeing you eat, you aren't putting on a show; you're making a conscious decision to shift your habits. Shifting your habits isn't what you do to cover up the fact that you are not yet in the healthiest place with your body image—it's an essential part of the work that will get you where you want to be. Your child needs to know that you are on that road and you intend to stay there.

"Our feelings about our bodies are habitual. If we habitually are kind and respectful and appreciative of them, they will serve us and we'll feel good about them. If we trash them, misuse them, abuse them with vicious criticism—we'll feel bad about them," says Tracee, thirty-five.

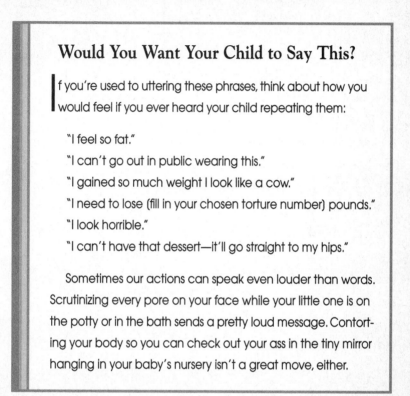

Would You Want Your Child to Say This?

If you're used to uttering these phrases, think about how you would feel if you ever heard your child repeating them:

"I feel so fat."

"I can't go out in public wearing this."

"I gained so much weight I look like a cow."

"I need to lose (fill in your chosen torture number) pounds."

"I look horrible."

"I can't have that dessert—it'll go straight to my hips."

Sometimes our actions can speak even louder than words. Scrutinizing every pore on your face while your little one is on the potty or in the bath sends a pretty loud message. Contorting your body so you can check out your ass in the tiny mirror hanging in your baby's nursery isn't a great move, either.

You can give your children food, but you can't really teach them to nourish themselves if you don't know how to nourish yourself. If you are unable to demonstrate what it looks like to make balanced food choices, to eat when you're hungry and stop when you're full, how can you possibly expect your children to learn? Does your child hear you talk about "bad" foods? Has your child ever seen you enjoy a sweet cupcake or an ice cream cone? Does she hear you say, "I'm hungry" and "I'm full"? Do your children feel a sense of family, community, and safety when you eat meals together, or are your guilt and anxiety unseen guests at the table? Do they understand that exercise isn't just for burning calories? Before we can pass along healthy attitudes about food and weight to our children, we have to embrace them for ourselves first. And we have to work for them.

Magali says:

"I try to give my three-year-old daughter choices, and that includes food choices. Dessert is a daily option for her after lunch and dinner. I don't buy junk food, but she has access to ice creams, sorbets, Tofutti Cuties, her own stash of chocolate, yogurt, and fruit. There are no 'bad' foods and nothing is forbidden. One day after lunch, I asked her if she wanted some chocolate. She shook her head firmly and asked for more lychees. My au pair was incredulous. 'Are you sure you don't want *chocolate?*' she nudged. My daughter knew what she wanted: 'No, thanks. More lychees, please.' To me, this is such a basic example of how taking the restriction away from food makes it more benign. I am happy that my daughter is learning to eat intuitively. That's something that took me a long time to learn for myself."

In Her Own Words:

The Power of Our Conversations

I have a daughter. It's really made me conscious of how everyone I know talks about their bodies. One thing I can do is not go on at length about my body and ask my friends to do the same. I want my daughter to have examples of women who don't pay attention to that.

Of course she's going to get out in the world and her friends are going to do it and I read these horror stories about very young girls going on diets and it's terrifying. I have to try, though. As I tell my friends not to talk about this stuff in front of her, they all start talking about their own mothers' attitudes toward their looks, and it's incredible! This stuff is handed down. Someone will remember that her mom was always calling herself fat and someone else talks about how her mom was tugging at her clothing. Of course, there's the really horrible level where the mom points out things that are wrong with the kid, but the secondary level is when moms point out things about themselves.

At the same time, when she does have body issues, I don't want her to feel that she can't come to me with them. I don't want her to think that she'll get shut down if she says she doesn't like how her butt looks. She should be able to say it. It's overwhelming, but then she's ten months old! So far so good. Maybe we'll just have a lot of conversations about it before she becomes a teenager and starts completely ignoring me. We'll go to movies and talk about women's bodies. I don't know. We'll see.

Amy, 37

We can't shield our children from all the conflicting messages about food, weight, and body image that are floating around out there. But we can try to change our own attitudes, behaviors, and conversations so they match the values we want our children to learn. We can teach our children how to be critical media consumers by talking to them about the difference between reality and retouching. We can give them the tools to understand and decode the business of celebrity media (see chapter 2, "Media Madness"). Even a simple request to stop body bashing can lead to deeper conversations among friends, who will think and learn, and pass it on. Let your positive actions lead the way. There is no prescribed road map, but we do know where you have to start—with yourself.

What Our Children Can Teach Us

Children put your life in perspective. You are still you—but the job you have as a parent is more important than anything you've ever done. There is love in your heart that you never imagined could be such a *force*. "Watching the birth of my daughter, seeing her in the flesh for the first time was the strongest love I have ever felt, love that was so instant and complete and pure," says Jeff, forty-two. "Then I got a closer look at her and got really scared because I wasn't sure if everything was the way it was supposed to be. Your life changes in ways that you would never be able to define without experiencing it firsthand." Those responsibilities and that overwhelming love can knock you off your feet and sometimes they can scare the crap out of you. You'll likely gain a deeper appreciation for what your own parents went through, and you might suddenly find yourself empathizing with their mistakes and shortcomings.

Reflecting on what it means to have a mother's body can help some women let go of the self-criticism they carried with them for all the years before they carried their babies. "I feel better about my body the more kids I have. It's less of a commodity now and more of a vessel," says Kristen, thirty-four. Tell your children that you appreciate your body because it brought them into the world instead of covering up in shame.

Even the process of watching your child's body grow can offer new insight into your own issues: "A really healing thing has happened with my daughter," says Lisa, thirty-five. "When I see her—I call her naked baby because she loves being naked—it's amazing to see her body. She's growing into my body shape. I love it so much in her. It's just making me love and accept it more in me."

Stop It, Supermommy!
How to Take Care of Ourselves and
Give Up the Quest for Perfection

Throughout pregnancy and after delivery, you might have a hard time turning down that insistent, nagging voice in your head—the one that keeps asking: *Am I doing this right? Is my baby passing all the right tests? Did I gain the right amount of weight? Will I lose it in the right amount of time? Do I have the right products? Did I choose the right hospital/doctor/midwife? Did I have the right delivery? Am I feeding/changing/holding my baby the way I should be?*

This is a whole new world, and it's normal to feel unsure of yourself—especially when those hormones are raging through your system and compounding the insecurities that are already brewing. But when perfectionism is your MO, you will have a very hard time feeling fulfilled as a mother.

Life is an endless stream of disappointments for mothers and mothers-to-be who are trying to be perfect. Your pregnancy and delivery might not go the way you dreamed. You will make mistakes as a mom. You will say things you regret and you will make decisions you wish you could take back. You will let yourself get too exhausted from time to time and you'll lash out at your partner, your kids, even yourself. You will never be exactly the supermommy you strive to be because there will always be one more thing you could do better, five more pounds you could lose, ten more minutes you could spend working on that presentation, or twenty more reps you could do at the gym.

Dos and Don'ts for Recovering Super Mommies

DO move on from your mistakes and figure out what you will do differently next time.

DON'T ruminate over all the couldas and shouldas and declare yourself the Worst Mommy in the World.

DO teach your kids that it's okay to fall on their faces every once in a while, especially if those experiences help them learn.

DON'T counteract that important lesson by constantly avoiding anything in your life that might make you feel like a "failure."

DO help your child understand that women's bodies come in all shapes and sizes and no one is more "perfect" than anyone else.

DON'T beat yourself up if you're still trying to accept your own body. If you make it clear to your children that self-acceptance and respect are your goals, they will get it.

Pretty much every new mom we met talked about how emo-tionally and physically draining pregnancy and new motherhood can be. The rewards can be rich, but it's harder to appreciate them when you're putting extra pressure on yourself—on top of the basic exhaustion you'll already be experiencing.

"I'm a huge feminist. I've always believed in women's rights, but I had this false notion that you can have it all. And you can't," confesses Lisa, a thirty-five-year-old new mother. "I constantly feel unfulfilled. When I'm home with the baby, I want to be working. When I'm working, I want to be home with the baby. It's like you could have it all, but you just can't be good at everything."

It will be a challenge to balance the new responsibilities of motherhood with all the other parts of your life. Actress Bridget Moynahan, who has plenty of resources and extra help, says it wasn't easy for her to figure out. "It's almost like you're juggling life and you've got three balls in the air and somebody tosses you this big fourth ball and you have to carry that big new ball," she told us. "So how do you start throwing in these other pieces of your life while keeping everything moving smoothly? Some things just don't get put back in. You find out very quickly what things you can't handle and what things are important and what things aren't. I had to give respect to what that was and slowly start adding things to see how things would move. I had to do it at my pace. So many people say, 'Oh, you should be doing this' or 'You should be doing that' and it really had to be about how I wanted to do it and at my pace."

It's not our responsibilities as parents, partners, professionals, and individuals that make so many women feel overwhelmed and inadequate; it's the pressure super mommies feel—from the out-side world and from their inner critics—to do everything and be everything to everyone. We compare our bodies to those of other women; we compare our babies to other babies. We measure our waists and we track percentiles. We take on more than we can realistically handle and we lie awake at night fearing potential screwups or wondering what others think of our choices.

None of these worries and comparisons will make us better mothers. In fact, the tragic irony is that the women who try the hardest to do everything just right are the ones who are sending the wrong messages to their children about what true confidence and resilience really look like. Our children won't benefit from hearing us talk about how we're not good enough. They *will* benefit from hearing us advocate for balance and flexibility. They don't need to see us carrying the burden of perfection on our shoulders. They *do* need to see that we can take care of ourselves and give ourselves a break.

In Her Own Words:

The Lessons in "Imperfection"

My first son was born deaf and it devastated me. You do sud-denly start thinking people are going to say it's your fault, even though you know it's not your fault. It's this awful feeling. And then when my second son was born with an eye problem, I had that feeling even stronger. You feel like a fake. People had given me all these beautiful things. I remember looking at the crib with the bumper on and everything like that, and thinking, *It's fucked, you know, it's fucked because I got a baby with a gimpy eye.* That was in my darkest hour. Somebody comes up and says, 'Congratulations, you have a baby!" and you're like, "Thank you for the sweet beautiful blanket, but I fucked up, you know." And you can't help that feeling.

But I said *no* to the guilt. I was going to enjoy him for what he is right here and now. . . . We're taught as women that it's our God-given right to have babies. You want two? You want a boy, a girl? Go on, then, you can do anything you want. They're going to be happy, healthy, and they will look after you. It will be great. People take that for granted. It's not our right to birth children. It is, in fact, a miracle.

Hermione, 44

There is a lot of power in our "imperfections." For one thing, they unite us. If we've learned anything from writing this book, it's that all of us mothers and mothers-to-be are seriously flawed. We've got stretch marks and sagging skin and we've got deep fears and insecurities about how to teach our children to love their bodies when we haven't quite figured out how to love our own. We fear judgment from others, but we judge ourselves daily.

We heard the same frustrations over and over again from women whose lives couldn't have appeared more different on the surface. We are all struggling, and most of us are struggling as women so often do—alone and in silence.

We created the Healthy Beauty Pledge (page vii) to give every woman who reads this book a way to take these ideas from the page to her life as a mother. They are promises you make to yourself, but by signing your name, you are joining other women who understand what these pressures feel like—mothers and moms-to-be who, like you, are doing their best to find balance and confidence, and to love their bodies. This *is* a healthy beauty revolution. We're starting it together.

Acknowledgments

This book would not have been possible without the participation of hundreds of women who bravely shared their experiences and proved that as mothers and mothers-to-be, we can find tremendous power in honesty and imperfections.

Our tireless research assistant Sivan Kovnator transcribed interviews, tracked down resources, and made it possible for us to highlight so many women's voices in this book. We also thank Susan Brown for her willingness to dive into the transcripts.

Our literary agent Jacqueline Hackett believed in this project from day one and helped us find it the right home.

Trader Joe's: your tea and goat cheese sustained us through many all-day and late-night writing sessions. There might have been a few glasses of red wine in there, too.

We were fortunate to know Nance Mitchell, a bright and witty beauty guru who shared her expertise for this project. She will be missed.

Monica Martinez, Alvera Taheri, Martha Mysko, and Irene Shoikhet were kind enough to lend their creative talents to the visual elements of the book.

To Allison Janse, our brilliant editor, and all the other wonderful folks at HCI—we are so grateful to you for guiding this project and bringing our "baby" into the world.

Magali:

I would like to thank my daughter for making me a better person, my mother for being such a "grande dame," all my friends I dragged into this book who trusted me with their thoughts and sometimes their very intimate moments, and the others who supported and encouraged me through this process. And finally, the Mysko for continuing to share a vision and for creating this book with me—a work that I am most proud of.

I would like to dedicate this book to my father, who gave me the strength to be myself, the discipline to fulfill my dreams, the security to go beyond my fears, and the example of a parent I strive to be. I wish for him to be proud of me, as I am forever proud to have had the privilege to call him "mon papa."

Claire:

In writing a book about becoming a mother, I can't help but thank my lucky stars for my own mother, who is all-around fabulous and who has always nurtured the writer in me. I am also forever thankful for my husband, Joshua Brown (who now knows more about pregnancy and new motherhood than he could possibly have wanted to know), and my amazing family and circle of friends for their questions, curiosity, support, and encouragement. And of course I must thank my co-author and partner-in-crime Magali. It's been quite a journey. I'm looking forward to the next chapter.

Resources

General Pregnancy and Motherhood Resources

BabyCenter.com
Expert information and real-world advice for women at all stages—from trying to conceive to raising kids.

Babble.com
Blogs, articles, and community for parents and parents-to-be.

CaféMom.com
An online community where you can share and connect with other moms.

BlogHer.com
A network that includes many excellent parenting and pregnancy blogs written from diverse perspectives.

Momsrising.org
"Where moms and the people who love them go to change the world."

Singlemommyhood.com
Blog posts, articles, advice, and resources for single moms.

American Academy of Pediatrics
aap.org
The AAP website highlights the latest research and AAP recommendations on hundreds of children's health topics.

Berkeley Parents Network
Parents.berkeley.edu
Founded by a group of parents in the San Francisco Bay area, this website contains thousands of searchable pages of resources and advice, as well as newsletters on parenting topics.

Featured in this book:

Sherry Rumsey, doula, childbirth class instructor, and student midwife
BirthingBaby.com

Barbara Dehn, RN, MS, NP
Barbsdailydose.typepad.com

Lamaze International
Lamaze.org
Lamaze serves as a resource for information about what to expect and what
choices are available during the childbearing years. Their website offers referrals to local childbirth educators.

Body Image Resources

The Belly Project
Thebellyproject.wordpress.com
This project spotlights real women's bodies, focusing on what women's bellies
really look like before and after pregnancy.

Dove Self-Esteem Fund
Dove offers a wide variety of resources, tips, and tools for moms and mentors
who want to raise kids with healthy self-esteem.
Campaignforrealbeauty.com

Featured in this book:

Meredith Nash
Babybumpproject.blogspot.com
Dr. Meredith Nash's research focuses on how the media obsession with
celebrity pregnancy affects women. Her blog offers her reflections and opinions about the latest "baby bump" and "postbaby body" stories.

The Shape of a Mother
Theshapeofamother.com
This website was started by a mother who recognized that most women don't
see pictures of real pregnant or post-childbirth bodies, but we do see plenty of

airbrushed and "perfect" bodies in the media. Women submit their real (and unretouched) pictures, sometimes with accompanying blog posts about how they feel about their bodies.

Eating Disorders and Disordered Eating

The National Eating Disorders Association
nationaleatingdisorders.org
800-931-2237
NEDA operates a toll-free helpline and referral service (available by phone or on their website). Ask for help and find treatment and support groups in your area.

National Association of Anorexia Nervosa and Associated Disorders
Anad.org
ANAD hosts more than 200 support groups in the United States and a few in other countries.

Edreferral.com
This searchable database offers lists of local treatment options and articles on eating disorders.

Gurze.com
The most comprehensive catalog of eating disorder and body image books and resources available.

Featured in this book:

Cynthia Bulik, Ph.D.
UNCeatingdisorders.org

Lesley Goth, PsyD
lgcounselingservices.com

Breastfeeding

La Leche League International
1 800 la leche
www.llli.org

Find breastfeeding support, information, healthcare providers, and resources about your rights.

The Pump Station
Breast pumps and breastfeeding accessories, resources, and how-to videos
Pumpstation.com

Featured in this book:

Blacktating
Blacktating.blogspot.com
Breastfeeding news and views from a mom of color.

Formula Fed and Flexible Parenting
Flexibleparenting.com
A personal blog documenting one woman's adventures in formula feeding.

Beauty and Style Resources

Featured in this book:

Marlien Rentmeester, *Lucky* magazine
Luckymag.com

Summer Rayne Oakes, author of *Style, Naturally*
Summerrayneoakes.com

Jessa Blades, Founder of Blades Natural Beauty
Bladesnaturalbeauty.com

Alvera Taheri Photography
Alveraphotography.com

Fitness Resources

Babyfit.com
Expert exercise tips, FAQs, and information about fitness safety during pregnancy.

Featured in this book:

Teigh McDonough, Swerve Studio
swervestudio.com

Mary Powell, LillySerpentine Fusion Belly Dance
lillyserpentinefusionbellydance.com

Ramona Braganza, celebrity fitness trainer
www.ramonabraganza.com

To learn more about the authors, share your experiences, and join the healthy beauty revolution, go to healthybeautypledge.com.

Index

Note: Italicized page numbers followed by an *f* indicate figures or illustrations.

behavior, 128, 131
as fetal health risk, 151
during pregnancy, 136
recovery from, 145–146, 158,
206–207
support resources, 227
teens at risk, 210, 213
triggers, 148

R
Rentmeester, Marlien, 98–99, 228
Rochon-Vollet, Stephane, 40
Rumsey, Sherry
on breastfeeding, 171–172
on dealing with Oversharers,
181
on family drama, 193
on flexibility, 26
on partner participation, 77
on postpartum realities, 28–29,
79–80
website, 226

S
secret eating, 128
Self magazine, 127
self-care
beauty regimens, 90–92,
105–108, 118–123
postpartum, 117, 120–121
teaching by example, 131,
211–220
self-worth, 28, 50–52
sex
breastfeeding and, 86–87, 164
after childbirth, 78–86
intimacy, 61–62
libido, 65, 72–73, 86–87, 164
parenthood and, 61–62

during pregnancy, 61–66, 71,
76, 86
shame, 125–127, 139–142
Shape magazine, 54
Shape of a Mother website, 226
significant others. *see* partners
single mothers' resource, 225
Singlemommyhood.com, 225
skin problems, 113–114
smell, sense of, 114
Spears, Britney, 39
Spelling, Tori, 56
spouses. *see* partners
stereotypes, unrealistic, 136–138
stretch marks, 6, 112–113
style. *see* fashion/style
Style, Naturally (Oakes), 109, 228
style tips, 98–99, 116–117
supermommies, 217–222
superwoman syndrome, 148
support
from friends, 134
Sutter, Trista, 39
SWERVE Studio, 48, 229
swimming, 23

T
3-2-1 Baby Bulge Be Gone
program, 44–45
tabloids
celebrity baby timeline, 54–55
celebrity moms, 35–42, 54–55,
132
paparazzi, 40–41
Taheri, Alvera, 101–103, 228
teasing, 195–196
"Till Children Do Us Part,"
(Coontz), 87–88
top body fears, 4–5

About the Authors

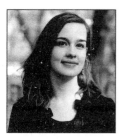

Claire Mysko is an internationally recognized expert on the issues facing women and girls today. As the director of the American Anorexia Bulimia Association, she oversaw outreach programs and managed the organization's hotline. She was the executive editor of SmartGirl and served as the assistant director of communications at Girls Incorporated, the organization that inspires all girls to be strong, smart, and bold. Her book for tween girls, *Girls Inc. Presents: You're Amazing! A No-Pressure Guide to Being Your Best Self*, was published by Adams Media in 2008. Claire has an MA in Gender Studies from the New School for Social Research. Her website (www.clairemysko.com) was recently named one of the top seven websites about "all things girl" by Shaping Youth.

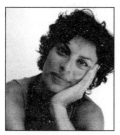

Magali Amadeï has appeared on the covers and pages of every major fashion magazine in the world, including *Vogue, Glamour, Marie Claire, Cosmopolitan, Elle,* and *Harper's Bazaar.* As a result of her battle with and victory over bulimia, Magali became the world's first top model to tour nationally and tell her story on behalf of an eating disorders organization. In 2005, she gave birth to a daughter. She appeared in *Sex and the City: The Movie*, and her essays are published in *Feeding the Fame* and *If I'd Known Then: Women in Their 20s and 30s Write a Letter to Their Younger Selves*.